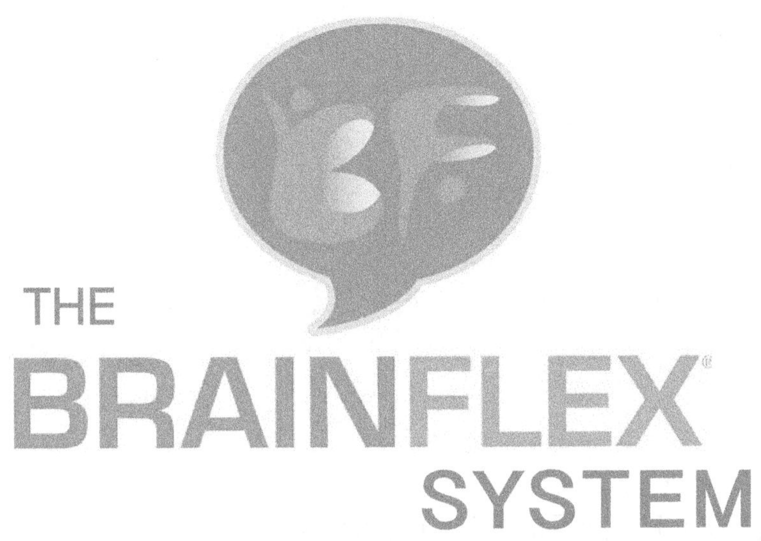

THE BRAINFLEX® SYSTEM

The Whole Person
Approach to Brain Health

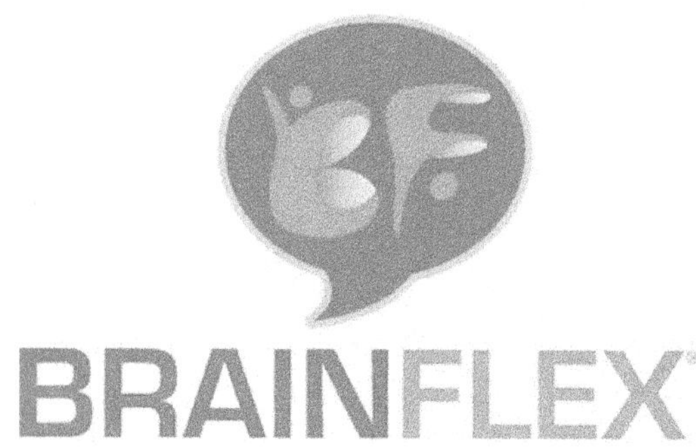

Volume 7 of 12 from 'The Prevention Series'
> *For those who want to be proactive against age related diseases, including those that cause cognitive impairment.*

www.brainflexwellness.com

Workbook Table of Contents

BRAINFLEX

Welcome to The BRAINFLEX System!

Congratulations! You've just taken another step in keeping your brain healthy for life!

The BrainFlex System makes maintaining the brain fun and easy. But don't be fooled by the fun! BrainFlex activities incorporate the lessons of medical research to keep the brain as healthy as possible while seniors age or face illnesses that impact the brain.

Each BrainFlex lesson includes 5 key components that work together to give the brain just what it needs each day to stay in top form.

Brain Exercise: Use it or lose it! Included in each of the 8 lessons are 3-5 brain stimulating exercises, all designed to stimulate various areas of the brain. Activities focus on creativity, problem solving, self-expression, brainstorming, etc., while others require a more structured focus requiring a more analytical or logical approach, and there are plenty of opportunities to exercise areas of the brain related to reasoning and math as well. Last, a life-long learning component (new information) is also incorporated into each workbook, which is designed to increase the brain's cognitive reserve.

Socialization: Whether seniors enjoy doing the workbook with others, or alone, our unique *'Discussion Sheets'* open the door for conversation at any time. Every lesson includes one BrainFlex *"News You Can Use"* sheet, focusing on a wide range of important topics, including the 'why' behind our BrainFlex concepts. Other topics include mental and emotional self-care, the importance of healthy sleep patterns, the impact of a positive mindset, healthy communication, tips on how to keep your relationships strong, and more! Each *'Discussion Sheet'* is designed to inform, educate, and encourage conversation.

Welcome to The BRAINFLEX System!

Nutrition: We are what we eat! Our goal is to stay mindful of the impact food choices have on the brain and body, as well as one's over-all well-being, and according to research, the healthier the gut, the healthier the brain. Four recipes are included in each workbook. Recipes are carefully selected and crafted for ease of preparation and enjoyment while eating! Nutritional information in the primary ingredients and specific benefits for the brain and body are listed with each recipe.

Physical Exercise/Meditation/Prayer:

Physical Exercise: Research tells us that physical activity is THE MOST IMPORTANT way to keep the brain healthy. Each workbook includes a monthly guide with detailed written and visual instructions, covering a variety of stretching and strengthening exercises. The goal of the exercise guide is to increase and/or maintain range of motion, strengthen the core and other vital muscles, increase oxygen flow and heart rate, (safely), and boost coordination, while reinforcing the brain-body connection.

Meditation/Prayer: Research confirms chronic stress ages the brain. It has also been shown that our 'mindset' impacts both the brain and body, making thinking and speaking positively vital to 'aging well'. Each BrainFlex workbook incorporates a variety of techniques, including breathing exercises, to help develop strategies to keep worry and anxiety away. Workbooks also include an instruction guide for prayer/meditation and a list of self-affirmations are included in each lesson.

To help seniors stay on track, workbooks in 'The Prevention' and 'Early-Mild' series' include a 'Personal Action Plan', which allows seniors to set monthly goals for each of the BrainFlex concepts. (Brain Stimulation, Socialization, Nutrition and Exercise w/Prayer and Meditation.) 'Wellness Notes' are provided to track the progress of each goal.

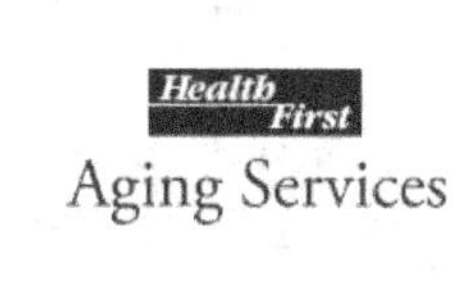

Aging Services

Health First Aging Services
Melbourne, FL

A NOTE FROM 'HEALTH FIRST' AGING SERVICES

My name is Pat DeAngelis and I am an RN, Licensed Nutrition Counselor and Patient/Caregiver Educator for Health First Inc. of Melbourne, Fl. I recently finished a five-week workshop for persons with Mild Cognitive Impairment using Workbook One of Early- Mild Series of the BrainFlex System. This was our first workshop using the BrainFlex system as an adjunct resource to provide continuity and continuous stimulation between group sessions. Our group averaged around twenty each week and met weekly, focusing on two lessons each week from the workbook along with an emphasis on one 'Healthy Lifestyle Habit' each week. A few exercises from the workbook were addressed as a group interaction activity during the two-hour session, however most of the exercises were reviewed and assigned for individual attention during the week at home. Physical Exercise, meditation, affirmations, action planning and journaling from the workbook were addressed each week.

The general feedback regarding the workbook was very positive. Several family members and friends of the MCI participants bought books for themselves and shared that they did see significant improvement in self-motivation, interest and focus from their loved ones. Some participants reported that, although they were overwhelmed with the various activities at the beginning, with encouragement and no pressure to finish every lesson each week, they did find accomplishments quite satisfying. I encouraged doing some activity daily and going back to do more or review as a good resource of brain stimulation after the workshop was completed.

As an educator I feel the workbook series is definitely a creditable resource to use as an interactive tool and provides the necessary activity for individuals to continue to implement the learned material into their daily lifestyle. Research has shown that developing and maintaining 'Healthy Lifestyle Habits' in all the areas addressed in the workbook series is extremely beneficial in managing and/or preventing all forms of Dementia.

Thank you, Melissa for all your research and professional knowledge that is demonstrated in your BrainFlex Series workbooks. Your work is extensive and a major community education resource for gaining and maintaining a healthy brain. Recent research has shown that with continuous attention to exercise, both physical and mental exercise, the brain can repair or bypass damaged areas of the brain to maintain desired functions for increased periods of time.

Pat DeAngelis RN, LNC

Caregiver Educator at Health First Aging Services Center For Family Caregivers.

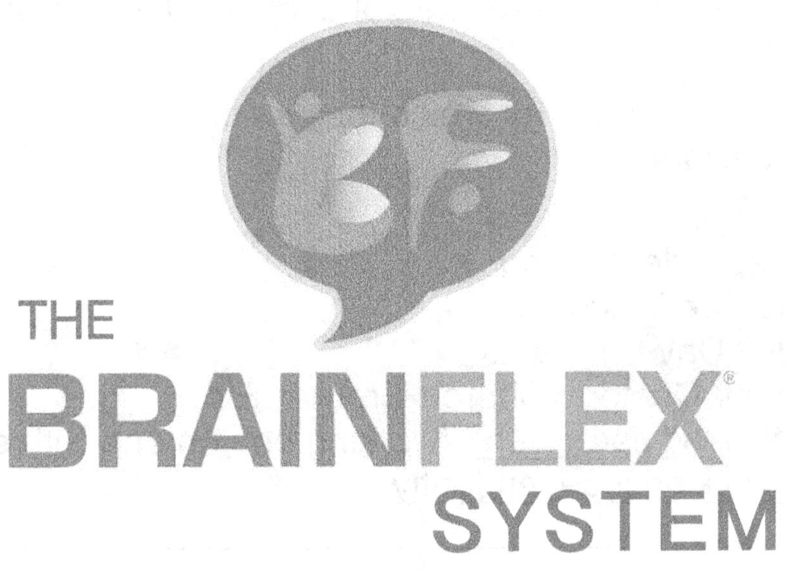

WORKBOOK GUIDE
This workbook is designed to be used in a variety of settings.

1. Small Groups
2. One on One
3. Individually

THE BRAINFLEX SYSTEM WORKBOOK GUIDE

The purpose of this guide is to help the user navigate through the workbook successfully, which will ensure everyone involved experiences the very best outcomes.

There are three categories for which the workbooks in the BrainFlex System were designed.

1. <u>Small Groups:</u>
   a. Independent Living
   b. Assisted Living
   c. Adult Day Programs
   d. Senior Centers, Church Groups, Etc.
2. <u>Family or hired caregivers</u>: (working one on one with seniors)
3. <u>Seniors working independently</u>

The BrainFlex System includes a three different series of interactive workbooks, each packed with brain stimulating activities that go beyond typical brain games and is the most comprehensive aging well program available in this format.

There are three levels in 'The BrainFlex System' series of workbooks.

1. The 'Prevention' Series
   a. This workbook series consists of volumes 1 through 12, with each workbook designed to last one month, (2 lessons per week), and is appropriate for the following:
      i. Anyone who would like to take a preventative (proactive) approach to aging well and brain health.
2. The 'Early ~ Mild' Series. (For those in the early stages of MCI)
   a. This workbook series consists of volumes 1 through 12, and is appropriate for those who have been experiencing dementia but can still understand and follow directions.
      i. Anyone experiencing mild memory loss but is determined to do all they can do to slow this process down.

      ii. Anyone who may be in the early stages of Alzheimer's or one of the other diseases that impacts brain function and would like to maintain their brain and/or slow the decline.

3. The 'Mid ~ Moderate' Series: For those w/Alzheimer's (and related diseases)

    a. This workbook series consists of volumes 1 through 12, with each workbook designed to last one month. (2 sessions/week) and is appropriate for those who may have been experiencing dementia for some time but can understand and follow basic directions with visual or verbal cuing.

The BrainFlex System has been developed for seniors committed to aging well, which is why each workbook is focused on 'the whole person'. This includes the brain, body, mind, spirit, emotions, and relationships. According to research, engaging in activities that contribute to the health of these areas is what gives seniors the best chance to maintain independence. Each concept of the BrainFlex program encourages seniors to be proactive against age related diseases, including Alzheimer's. 'The BrainFlex Workbook' equips seniors with the tools needed to age well.

The interactive lesson plans are designed to be completed in one month, (2 lessons each week). Each lesson takes 2 to 3 hours to complete in a group setting, and about 1 ½ to 2 hours if done alone or with one other person.

NOTE: Sessions can be broken up into 2, 3 or 4 smaller sessions throughout the day or completed in one fun-filled session. *(i.e. Exercise @ 9am, Brain Stimulating Activities @ 11am, Interactive Nutrition @ 2pm and Meditation/Prayer with Self-Affirmations @ 7pm)* With that being said, our experience doing this live is that seniors enjoy the 2½ to 3 hour sessions.

KEEP IN MIND:
It's important to complete each worksheet in the lesson, rather than skipping around to find the activity that's most enjoyable. Although we understand this temptation ☺, it will not provide exercise to every area of the brain. As a matter of fact, the activities you enjoy the least are likely to be the most beneficial to your brain.

Both The Preventative Series and The Early ~ Mild Series of workbooks include a 'Personal Action Plan'. This plan is created by the individual, (although family members and/or caregivers may also want to contribute), and is based on the four concepts that have been shown to contribute the most to 'Aging Well' and to help slow down cognitive decline. Two goals are created for each of the <u>concepts</u> on which the BrainFlex program is built. *(See these concepts on the following page.)*

BrainFlex Concepts

1. Social |Connections
2. Nutrition
3. Brain Stimulating Activities
4. Physical Exercise with Meditation

(A positive mindset and healthy sleep patterns are also key to aging well and discussed frequently throughout the workbooks.)

Tracking your Monthly Personal Action Plan:
Steps taken to meet goals on the personal action plan can be tracked on the weekly 'Wellness Journal' pages, found in the back of each workbook in the 'Preventive' and 'Mild/Early' series'. The 'Personal Action Plan' and the 'Wellness Notes' are wonderful tools for families and primary care physicians.

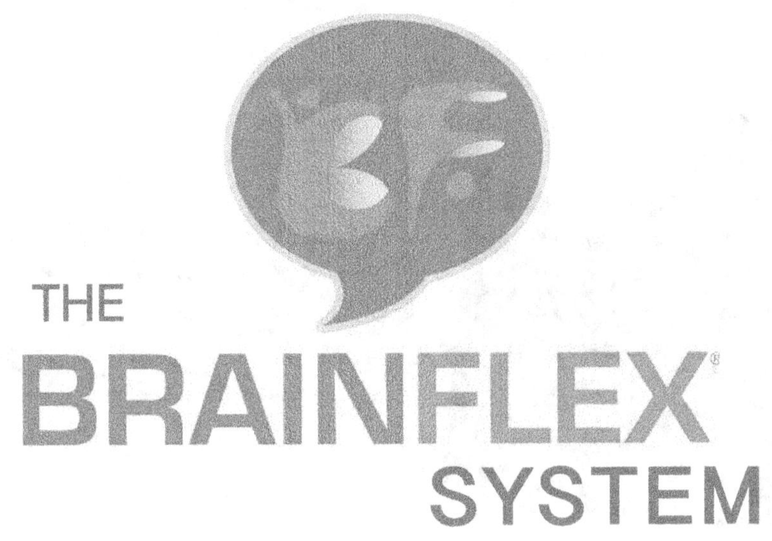

THE BRAINFLEX® SYSTEM

EXERCISE GUIDE

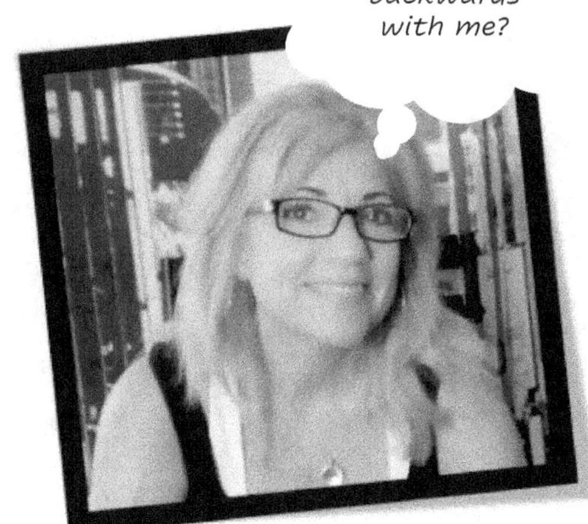

Exercise Series

You should always speak to a doctor before you change, start or stop any part of your healthcare plan, including physical activity or exercise.

Also, be sure to speak with your doctor before exercising if the following are applicable to you:

1. A long period of inactivity
2. Recent hospitalization
3. Recent surgeries

Stop and call 911 if you experience the following:

1. Unexplained shortness of breath
2. Pain in your neck, shoulders or arms
3. Leg pain, with or without swelling or tenderness
4. Dizziness
5. No one knows your body like you, so be sure to report anything that feels abnormal or unusual

IMPORTANT REMINDERS:
1. Form is very important. Be sure to keep your core tight, as if you are pulling your belly button back towards your spine.

2. Unless the exercise specifically instructs otherwise, keep your chin up, your shoulders back, and ensure your spine is as straight as possible. *(Avoid doing anything that causes you pain.)*

3. If at all possible, avoid using the back of the chair for support during exercise. Doing so will keep you from engaging your core, which is **KEY to balance.**

4. Take breaks when necessary, and be sure to drink plenty of water, before...during and after exercise.

Neck Stretch

Counting to 10, slowly begin to tilt your head so the ear is over the shoulder as shown below. Follow the visual guide, hold for 5 seconds and count to 10 as you raise your head back to the starting position.
Repeat the stretch on the opposite side.

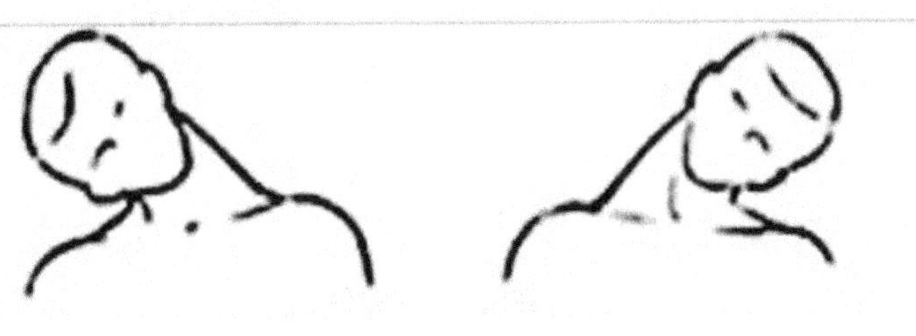

Reminder:
Refrain from doing anything that causes pain.

Hand, Finger and Arm Stretches

Follow the visual guide to begin stretching the muscles in your arms, hands & fingers, very gently. While counting to 10, gently lift the arms gently above the head.
(It's okay if you aren't able to lift arms straight up.)

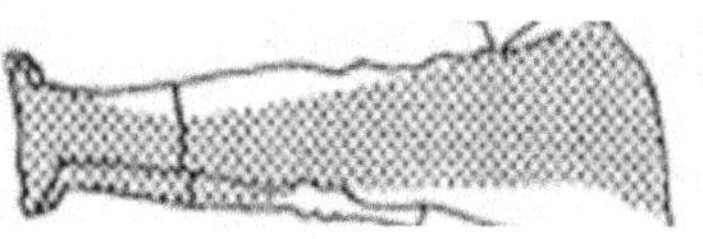

While counting to 10, slowly bring the arms back down,
then repeat for one more stretch.

__Reminder__: Refrain from doing anything that causes pain.

The Shoulder Shrug

Follow the visual guide to begin slowly stretching your neck and shoulder muscles, very gently.

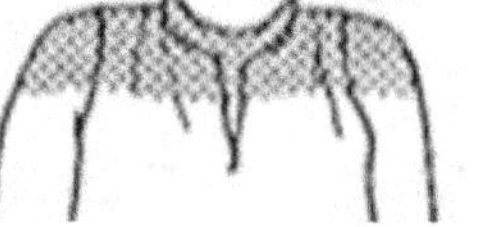

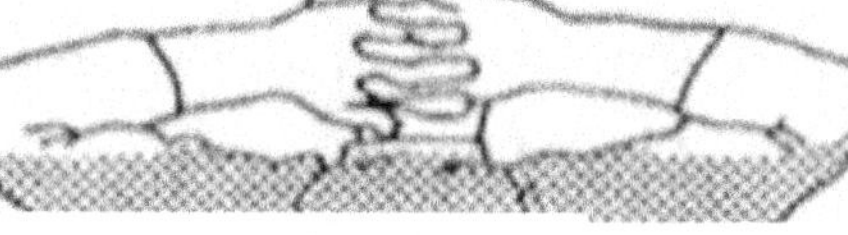

The Pectoral Stretch

Complete a total of 8 shoulder shrugs and
1 pectoral stretch,
(If you're able to do so.)

Waist and Core Exercise

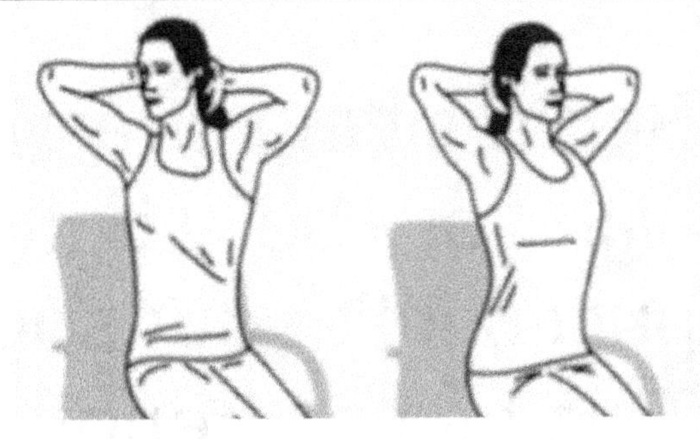

With your feet together on the floor, place your hands behind your head. *(if comfortable)* Slowly turn toward the right, twisting at the waist, then return to the starting position, and repeat, twisting to the left.

Complete 10 sets.

Thigh Exercises

Begin with a nice and tight core, shoulders back, and chin up.

Lift the right leg, until it's completely extended, hold for 10 seconds.

Repeat with opposite leg.

Complete one set of 8. (8 lifts on each side.)

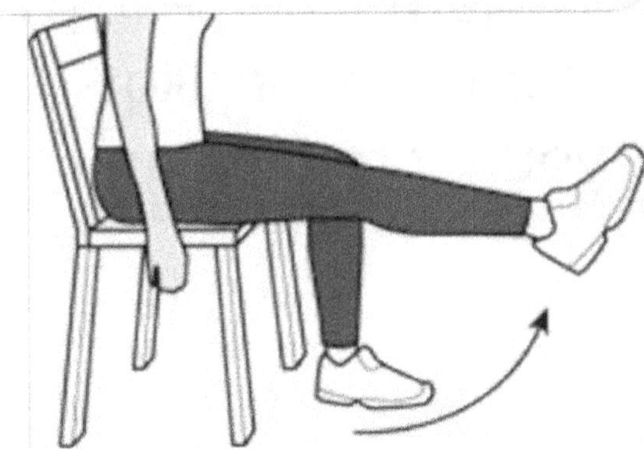

Begin sitting straight up, with your belly button pulled into your spine. This helps strengthen the core.

This exercise includes 4 slides with written and visual instructions. This is slide 1 of 4.

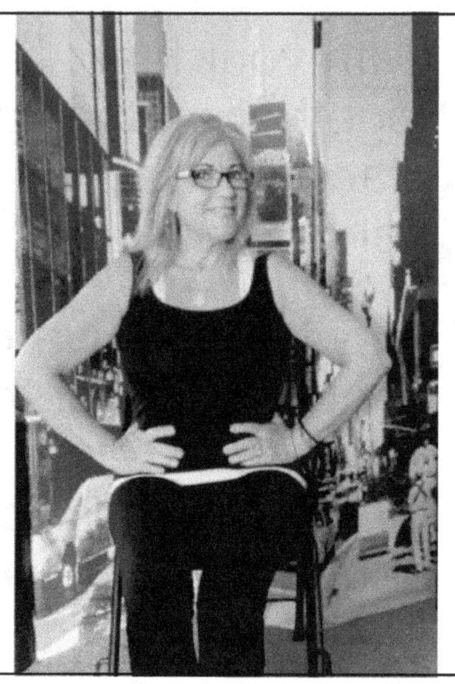

Start the exercise by lifting one knee straight up (towards the ceiling), Remembering to keep your core nice and tight...

Slide 2 of 4

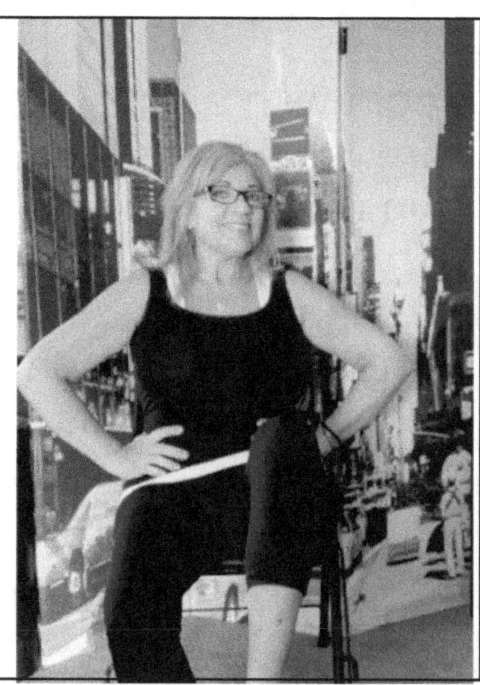

Continue by lifting the leg up, over and out, then barely tap the toe, before lifting the leg straight up and back to the starting position.

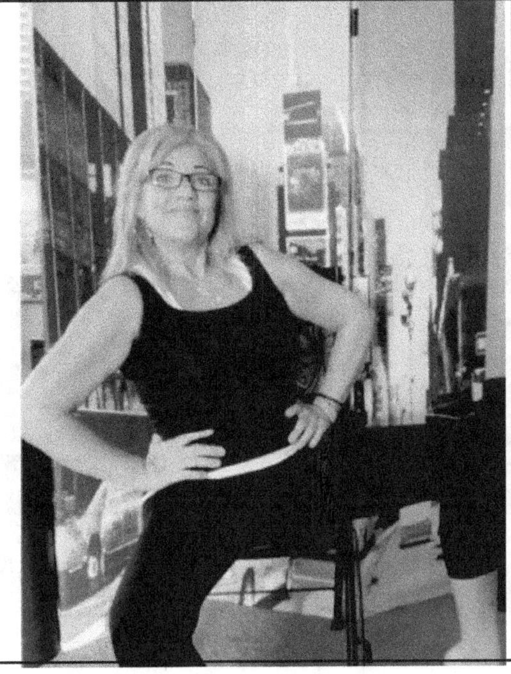

Slide 3 of 4

Once you return to the starting position,
(as if you were lifting your leg over a fire),
do the same exercise on the opposite leg.

Alternate legs,
24 repetitions.
(12 on each side.)

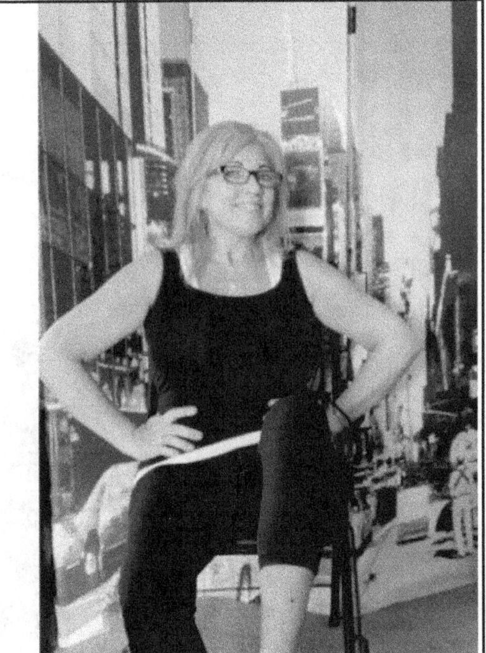

Slide 4 of 4

Arm Exercises

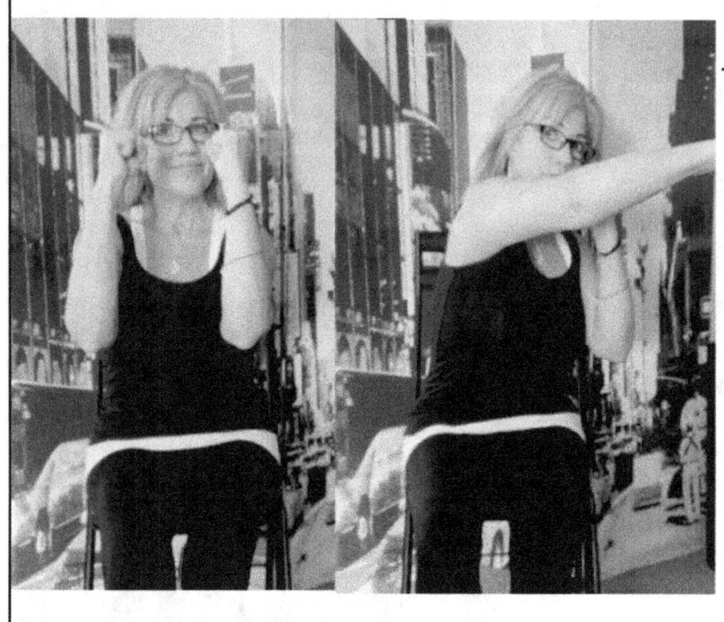

<u>Cross Body Jab (1 of 2)</u>

Plant your feet, and place your arms in a 'guarded' position.

Begin with a cross body jab using your right arm. Be sure to include a slight twist at the waist. Quickly return to the starting position.

(continued below)

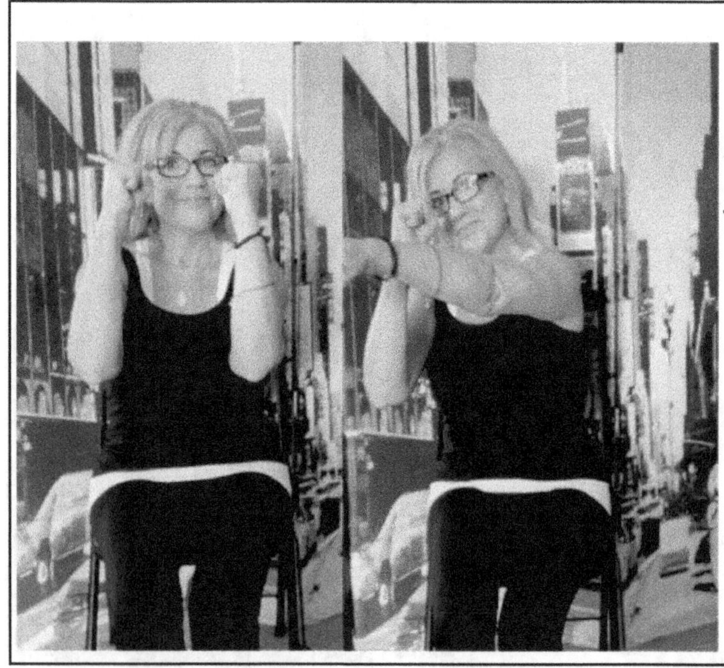

(2 of 2)

From the starting position, continue with the left arm, alternating arms with a cross body jab until you've completed 24.
(12 jabs with each arm.)

*Add some upbeat music to make this more challenging.
(and more fun too!)

Bicep Curls

<u>Written Instructions:</u>
Begin with your arms by your side, using a weight that is safe and comfortable for you, and okay with your doctor as well.

With palms facing out, bend your arms at the elbow, bringing the weights up to the position shown below.

Return to the starting position and repeat.
Complete a total of 12 bicep curls.

Working the Biceps

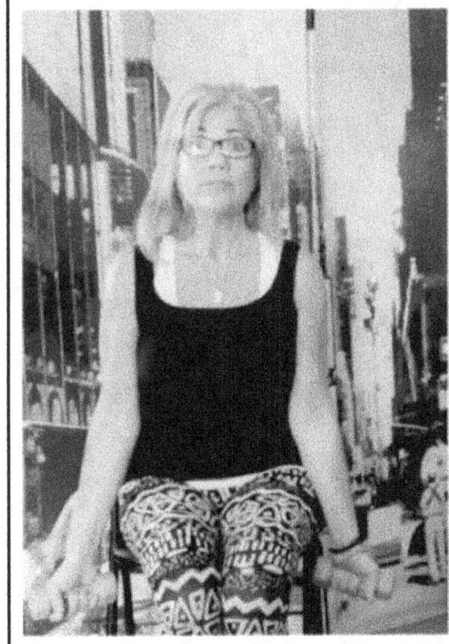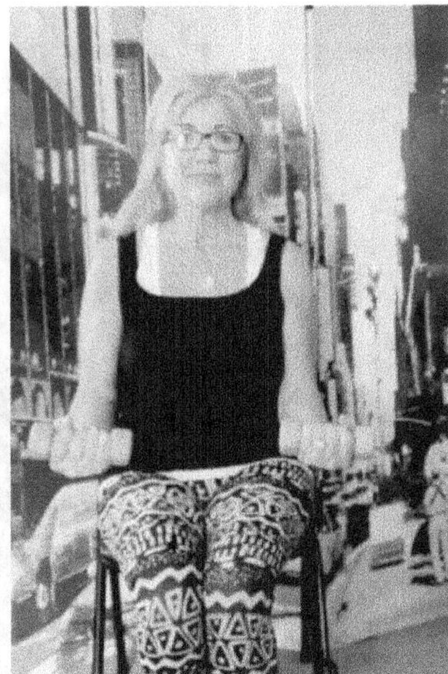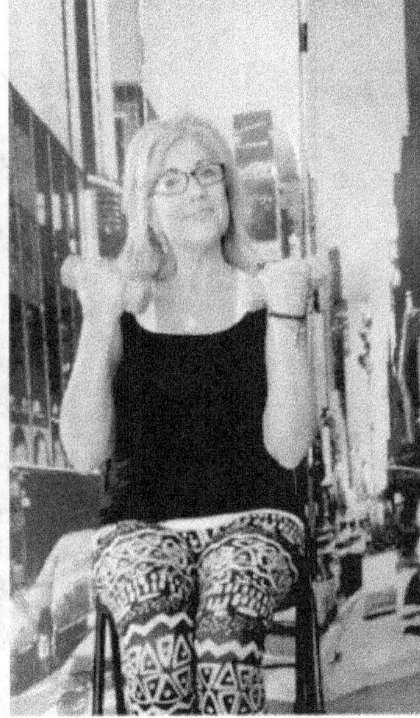

Triceps

**(One arm at a time)
Begin in the starting position, with your
palm facing inward, as shown.
Moving the arm from the elbow down only,
extend the arm backwards as shown, until the
bottom of your weight is facing the ceiling.
Return to starting position.
Complete 12 on each side.**

Working the Triceps

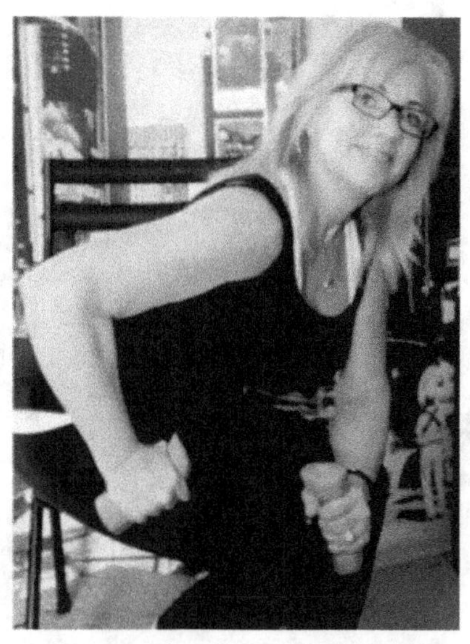
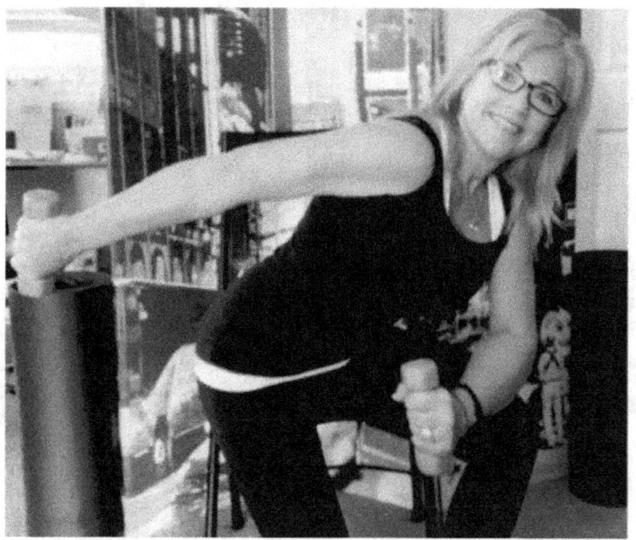

Side Stretches

In a seated position, place your feet flat on the floor,with your arms at your side and fingertips facing the floor. Begin with the right arm, (palm facing up), lift the right arm straight up, then over, until your fingertips are at 1:00. (Hold chair with opposite hand to keep balance if needed.) Return to the starting position and repeat on the other side, (11:00), for a total of 10 stretches.
(5 stretches on each side.)

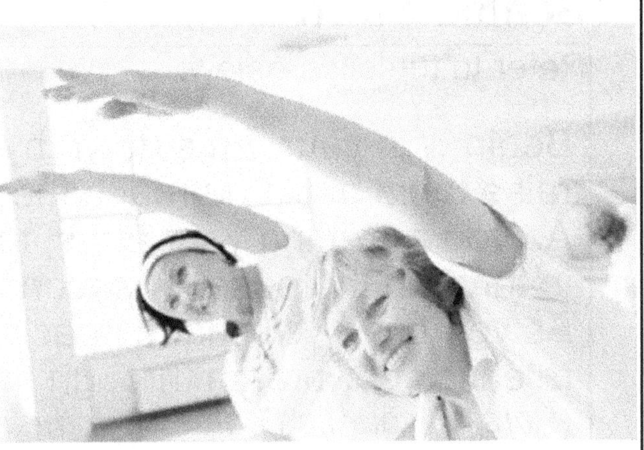

Inhale in through nose and exhale through the mouth with each stretch.

Arm Stretch

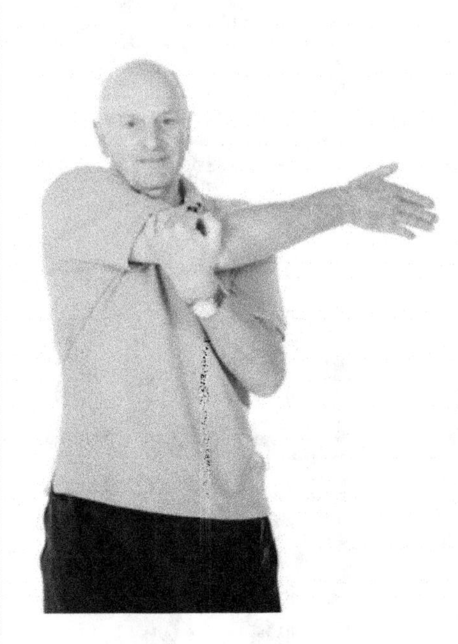

Begin with one arm straight out in front of you. Slowly move the arm across your body.
Place the opposite hand on your elbow, while gently pressing your arm in towards your body for a deeper stretch.
Hold for 10 seconds, then repeat on the opposite side.

For an optimal stretch, do your best to keep your shoulders as squared as possible.

Seated Stretch

Refer to the slide below.

Begin with your arms down by your side, and slowly
raise them until you reach the position shown.
As you are lifting your arms, take a deep breath,
in through the nose. (4 seconds)
As you bring your hands back down to your side,
release your breath through the mouth. (8 seconds)
(*Pursing your lips helps slow the release of breath.*)

Repeat this three times.

This is a great time to practice gratitude. Allow a few things for which you
are thankful to be seen by your mind's eye as you breathe in and out.

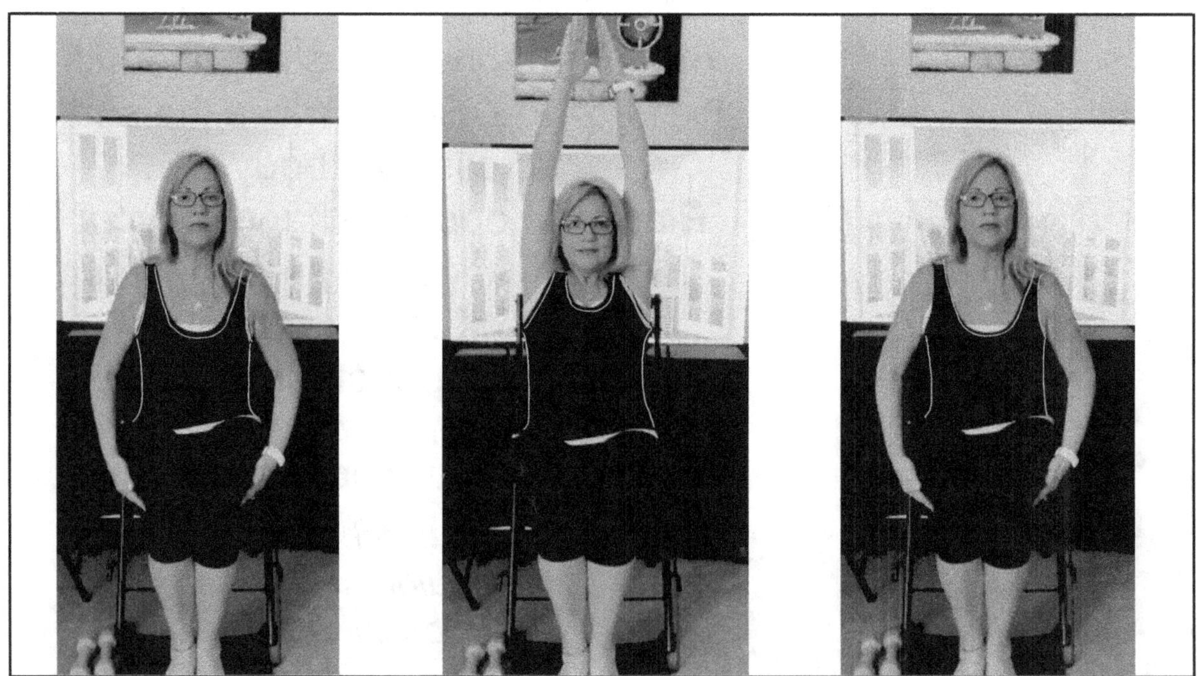

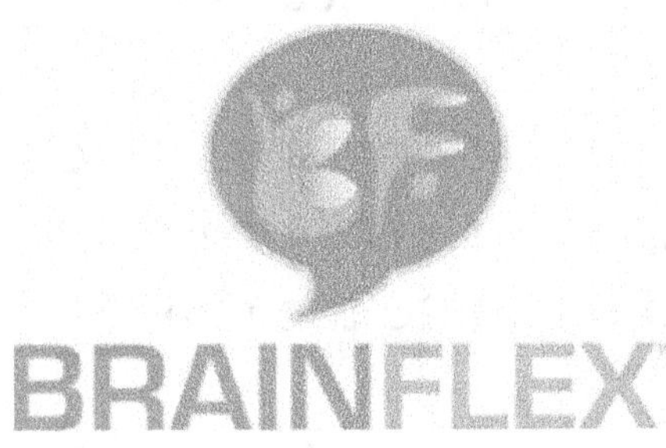

Prayer/Meditation Guide

Monthly Meditation/Prayer
Purposeful Breathing Guide
(Use w/Self-Affirmations Sheets)

Begin to play soft relaxing music. (Nature, Spa, Classical, etc.)

1. Get comfortable – Relax in a comfortable chair. Breathing in through the nose (this should take 4 seconds) then…out through the mouth, which should take about 8 seconds.
(Pursing your lips will help lengthen the time of the exhale.)
(*Repeat this breathing exercise once more.*)

2. Next, begin to relax the face muscles, (mouth, jaw), then relax the neck, shoulders, arms, hands, fingers, legs, feet, toes, and spine… letting yourself melt into the chair.

3. To begin, focus on the music while maintaining regulated breathing, [**Regulated Breathing**: *In through the nose and out through the nose, at a very steady pace, feeling the breath going in through your nose and out through your nose, noticing your belly rising and falling with each steady breath.*]

4. Next, focus on **gratitude. Thoughts of thankfulness**, allowing the people, places, things, etc., for which you are thankful to play over and over in your mind like a beautiful slide show. Focus on the word, 'Thank you'. (Hear it…say it…feel it, alongside your thoughts of gratitude.)

5. After a few minutes, focus back on the music and take two nice deep breaths (as instructed in #1), then settle back into your chair, once again, relaxing each muscle. (as instructed in #2)

BrainFlex® Wellness

Monthly Meditation/Prayer
Purposeful Breathing Guide
(Use w/Self-Affirmations Sheets)

6. Choose an affirmation from your 'Self-Affirmations' sheet, and repeat the affirmation out loud, then, as you listen to the music, focus on the words you just spoke, repeating them both out loud, and in your mind, as you practice your regulated breathing and relax to the music.

7. After a few minutes, choose a second affirmation from your 'Self-Affirmation' sheet, and repeat the process again, just as you did in #6.

8. After a few more minutes, choose a third affirmation from your 'Self-Affirmation' sheet, once again, repeating the process, just as you did in #6 & #7.

9. When you feel you are ready, place your focus back on the music and take two nice deep breaths, (following the instructions in #1), then settle back into your chair, relaxing each face muscle again, (as instructed in #2). When you are finished, return to your regulated/rhythmic breathing, (#3)

10. After a few minutes, return your focus back to gratitude and thankfulness. Once again, focusing on those things for which you are thankful...see them with your mind, as you hear the word, 'Thank You', playing over and over in your thoughts.

11. Before you finish, spend some time in prayer.

12. As you finish this time, repeat #1, taking 2-3 nice deep breaths.
   (Take your time getting up. Make sure to drink plenty of water.)

BrainFlex® Wellness

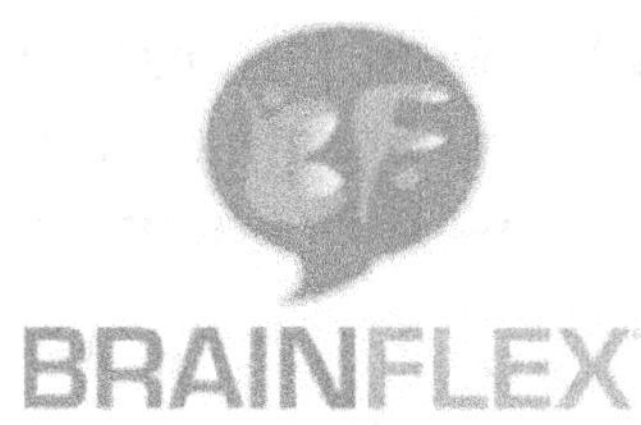

Gratitude.

Take a few minutes to pause and write down some things for which you are thankful.

____

____

____

____

____

____

____

____

____

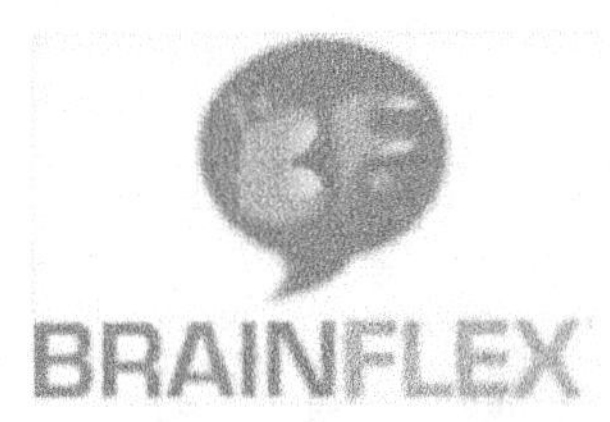

Week One
NUTRITIONAL RECIPE

Contributing to a
healthier brain & body

The health benefits in the recipe's ingredients will vary with each individual and depend heavily upon each person's level of commitment to making healthy life-style choices on a consistent basis.

BRAIN HEALTHY TRAIL MIX

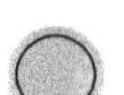

INGREDIENTS · SERVINGS: 4

¼ cup of raisins
¼ cup of dried cranberries
¼ cup of organic granola
¼ cup of cashews
¼ cup of pecans
¼ cup of walnuts
¼ cup of almonds
¼ cup of mini chocolate chips
(sweetened w/stevia)

HEALTH BENEFITS ~ ALMONDS...

PACKED FULL OF NUTRIENTS AND ARE
ESPECIALLY HIGH IN VITAMIN E

CONTAIN HEALTHY FATS NEEDED FOR
BRAIN HEALTH

LOADED WITH ANTIOXIDANTS, WHICH
FIGHT CELL DAMAGING FREE RADICALS

CAN HELP CONTROL BLOOD SUGAR LEVELS
AND LOWER LEVELS OF BAD CHOLESTEROL

HEALTH BENEFITS OF RAISINS

A Good Source of Fiber: Aids the digestive process

**A Good Source of Iron: Needed for red blood cell
production and to carry oxygen to other cells**

**Contains Calcium & Boron: Boron works w/
Calcium and Vitamin D to help keep our bones and
joints healthy.**

**Contains Antimicrobial Compounds:
Phytochemicals such as oleanolic acid and linoleic
acid, fight bacteria in the mouth that cause
cavities and gum disease.**

<u>**HEALTH BENEFITS: PECANS**</u>
**PECANS CONTAIN HEALTHY FATS AND ARE A GREAT
SOURCE OF PROTEIN. THE BENEFITS THEY PROVIDE ARE
NUMEROUS, BUT HERE ARE JUST A FEW...
->PROMOTE CARDIOVASCULAR HEALTH
->ASSIST WITH DIGESTIVE HEALTH
->PROMOTE HEALTHY BONES & TEETH
AND ALSO...**

HELPS REDUCE INFLAMMATION AND BLOOD PRESSURE

HEALTH BENEFITS: DRIED CRANBERRIES

Contains bioactive compounds: quinic, malic, & citric acids, which fight degenerative & chronic diseases

Beneficial to both the cardiovascular & immune systems

Helps maintain a healthy urinary tract

Rich in the antioxidants associated with reducing cholesterol

Can help prevent gum disease & stomach ulcers

Promotes healthy blood clotting & boosts metabolism

HEALTH BENEFITS: CASHEWS

- High in protein, providing that 'full feeling', which can help reduce the urge to snack.

- Protein contributes to healthy muscles

- Research has shown that cashews benefit both nerve and muscle function

- Contains heart-healthy mono-unsaturated fats
  - These essential fatty acids lower levels of bad cholesterol (LDL) while increasing levels of good cholesterol (HDL)

HEALTH BENEFITS: WALNUTS

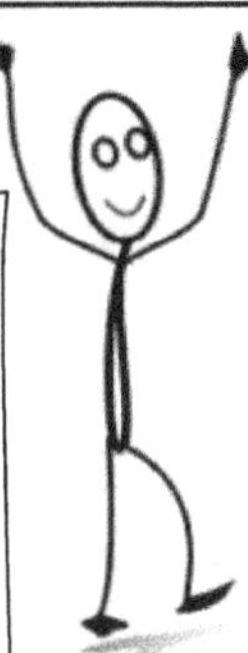

Omega-3's found in walnuts have been shown to...
  - **help battle symptoms of depression**
  - **promote a healthy gut, which has been shown to improve an individual's over all feeling of wellness**
  - **assists with weight control, due to the high levels of protein**
  - **provide the brain and body with a super plant source of Omega 3's**

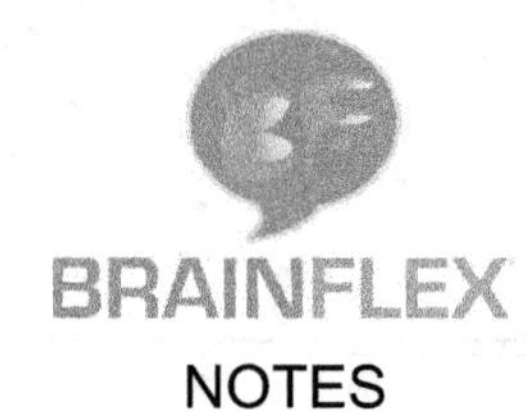

NOTES

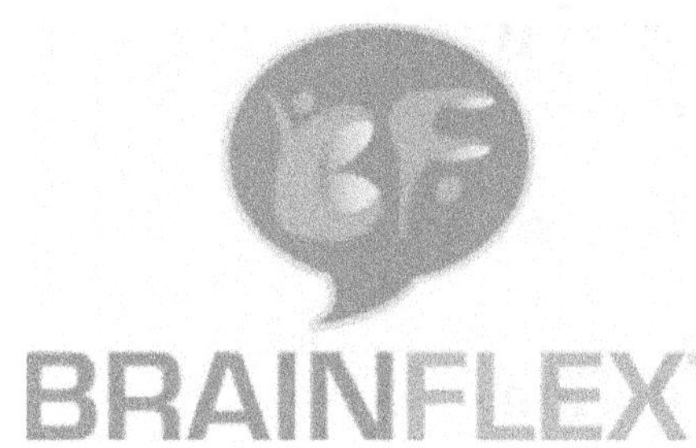

Lesson
1

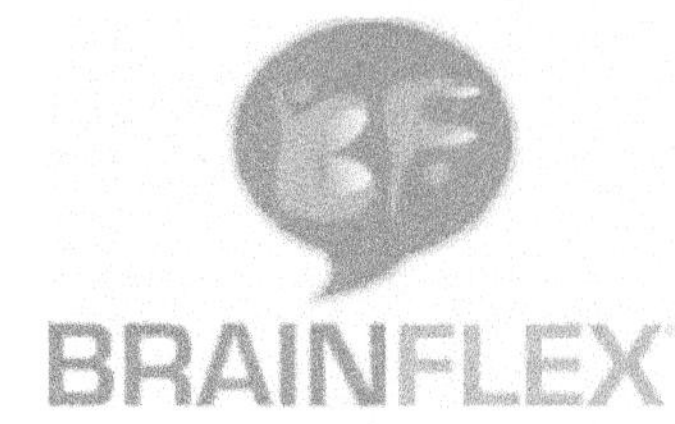

Reminder Page

Don't forget to check off the following after you complete them today:

_____ Exercise

_____ Prayer/Meditation

_____ Self-Affirmations

The self-affirmations included in our workbooks are built on a healthy love of self, not an egotistical kind of love. This portion of the Aging Well program is about self-respect, knowing that you are worthy… that you are good enough…just the way you are.

It's important to say each affirmation several times out loud, even if you aren't sure you believe what you're saying. Over time, your mind's eye will begin to see the world, (this includes YOU)…in a more positive light. We believe that we're all God's creation and that it's important to Him that we love and appreciate the unique design of every person, (this includes YOU).

I am beautiful…just the way I am.

I respect myself.

I am confident in who I am.

I let go of all negative thinking.

I will replace negative thoughts with positive ones.

<u>**LESSON 1: RESEARCH & DISCUSSION**</u>
(News you can use, and it makes for some great discussion too!!)

Brain Stimulating Activities Contribute to Brain Health

How often do you engage in activities that require math and logic? To many people, math and logic seem difficult, therefore, they try to avoid it as much as possible.

It's important to note that activities which require the use of math and logic provide an excellent workout for the brain. In addition, many research studies show that this type of mental stimulation, on a regular basis can even help prevent or slow down cognitive decline. One research study published in the New England Journal of Medicine, showed reduced systems of dementia in those who engaged in brain stimulating activities on a daily basis. (By 63%!)

According to the research, any type of brain challenge done on a daily basis can improve brain function, memory and even the capacity to reason.

Activities that incorporate math and logic, regardless of your age, provide an immense amount of exercise for the brain.

Last, learning new information is a wonderful way to stimulate brain cell growth and build the brain's cognitive reserve. A few examples are, learning a new language, studying a new subject, or learning how to play an instrument.

Building the brain's cognitive reserve provides resistance, or resilience, to deterioration in the brain. This idea first received significant consideration in the late 1980's, during 'The Nun Study', when researchers discovered that those participants in the study with the highest cognitive reserves were less likely to display symptoms of dementia, even if they were diagnosed with a disease that included dementia as a primary symptom, such as Alzheimer's.

WorksCited
Boomers w/Elderly Parents Engaging in Math-Games. (2017, August
6). Retrieved from Boomers with Elderly Parents:
http://www.boomers-with-elderly-parents.com/math-games.html

Brainagrams
Rearrange the letters in each underlined word in order to answer the questions below. Number one has been done for you as an example.

1. Steve and Robin went to the ***CINEMA*** to see the new movie,
    " **ICEMAN**" (*Hint: Freezing - Male*)

2. Sheri is happily ***MARRIED*** to Kevin, but she recently discovered
    that she has a secret ________________.
    (*Hint: When someone is attracted to you…*)

3. Nick bought three ***ACRES*** of land in Alaska so he could have snow
    mobile __________ on his property. (*Hint: On your mark…*)

4. Grandma always ***PATS*** her leg and _________ her foot when she
    hears music. (*Hint: Do this to keep the beat w/your feet.*)

5. Debby ***ATE*** a chocolate chip muffin, then said she still wanted to
    _______ a piece of cake. (*Hint: Present tense.*)

6. Many very well-known ***ACTORS*** are happy to __-________
    with other famous actors. (*Hint: Sharing the stardom.*)

7. Barney starred in a ***LIVE*** TV broadcast of what used to be a stage
    play called 'The _________ Brother.' (*Hint: Opposite of good.*)

8. When Don participated in his high school spelling bee, he
    misspelled ***ANGLE*** and instead, spelled ____________. (*Hint: Halo*)

9. Glenna loves to ***HEAR*** her pet _________ chomp on carrots.
    (*Hint: Usually larger than a rabbit.*)

10. Bud tried to teach his ***TEENAGER*** how to __________________
    more revenue on his paper route.
    (*HINT: To cause something to come about or to produce energy.*)

Associated Words-Language Center

From the list of words provided, choose the word that connects to the word before and to the word after. The first one is already completed as an example.

1. Year ____**Book**____ -> ____**Worm**____ -> ____**Wood**____ - ____**Pecker**__
    Worm   Pecker   Book   Wood

2. Heavy __________ -> __________ -> __________ -> __________
    Book   Rain   Check   Keeper

3. Pain __________ -> __________ -> __________ -> __________
    Killer   Line   Drive   Bee

4. Table __________ -> __________ -> __________ -> __________
    Shade   Lamp   Tree   Branch

5. Feeling __________ -> __________ -> __________ -> __________
    Blue   Light   Sky   Switch

6. Men's __________ -> __________ -> __________ -> __________
    Study   Case   Suit   Hall

7. Cold __________ -> __________ -> __________ -> __________
    Shoulder   Lady   Bug   Bag

8. Come __________ -> __________ -> __________ -> __________
    Stop   Sign   Back   Door

Create your own below:

______________ -> ______________ -> ______________ ->
______________ -> ______________

TRIVIA 'LOVE'

1. When you see 'XO' written in a love letter, what are they meant to represent?   **a. The Cross and an Egg**

   b. A Kiss and a Hug   **c. Sign Here**

2. Cupid has what name in Greek mythology?

   a. Satinous   **b. Eros**   **c. Cupidous**

3. In Greek mythology, who is Cupid's mother?
   a. Venus   **b. Marsa**   **c. Ethos**

4. In Greek mythology, with whom does Cupid fall in love?   **a. His own Psyche**

   b. His Aunt Ethel   **c. His 5th cousin**

5. Who was the legendary Benedictine monk who invented champagne?   **a. Steven Sweetheart**

   b. Dom Perignon   **c. Arnold the Great**

6. When did Sweethearts first get their shape?
   a. 1801   **b. 1901**   **c. 2001**

7. "Wearing your heart on your sleeve" has origins from honoring which Roman goddess?
   a. Muon   **b. Juno**   **c. Luno**

8. A single red rose surrounded by baby's breath is called what by florists?
   a. A Signature Bouquet   **b. A Signature Rose**

   c. A Signature Breath

TRIVIA 'LOVE'

9. In the Victorian era, mean-spirited Valentine's Day cards were called "_______________ Valentines."
   a. Vinegar   **b. Vile**   **c. Dark**

10. From where was the oldest-known Valentine's Day message sent?
    a. Church   **b. Prison**   **c. Unknown**

11. Who wrote the oldest-known Valentine's Day message?
    a. The Duke of Earl   **b. The Duke of Orleans**
    C. Dukes of Hazard

12. In what century was the oldest-known Valentine's Day message written?
    a. 1400's   **b. 1900's**   **c. Unknown**

13. About how many roses are sent on Valentine's Day each year?
    a. One million   **b. 15 million**   **c. 50 million**

14. Who invented the first Valentine's Day candy box?
    a. **Richard Cadbury**
    b. **Richard Nixon**
    c. **Willie Wonka**

15. As of the year of 2020, on average, how many marriage proposals are there on Valentine's Day?
    a. **Around 220**
    b. **Around 22,000**
    c. **Around 220,000**

Distributive Property: Simplify each equation below in box #1.
(Do your best to avoid looking at the answers shown in box #2.)

Box #1

$-4p(-3p - 4)$	$4h(-7 + 3h)$	$7x(-3x - 5)$
$2b(9b - 6)$	$2(6v - 1)$	$-3(-9 + 8r)$
$2k(-2 + 8k)$	$7n(-8n + 2)$	$2w(-6w - 1)$
$(7 + 2h)(-7)$	$-6d(4 + 5d)$	$(7 + 2h)(-7)$

ANSWERS

Box #2   Compare your completed equation with the answers provided.

$-4p(-3p - 4)$ $12p^2 + 16p$	$4h(-7 + 3h)$ $12h^2 - 28h$	$7x(-3x - 5)$ $-21x^2 - 35x$
$2b(9b - 6)$ $18b^2 - 12b$	$2(6v - 1)$ $12v - 2$	$-3(-9 + 8r)$ $-24r + 27$
$2k(-2 + 8k)$ $16k^2 - 4k$	$7n(-8n + 2)$ $-56n^2 + 14n$	$2w(-6w - 1)$ $-12w^2 - 2w$
$(7 + 2h)(-7)$ $-14h - 49$	$-6d(4 + 5d)$ $-30d^2 - 24d$	$(7 + 2h)(-7)$ $-14h - 49$

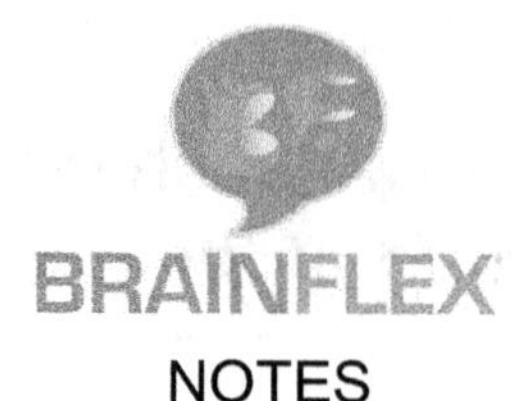

BRAINFLEX
NOTES

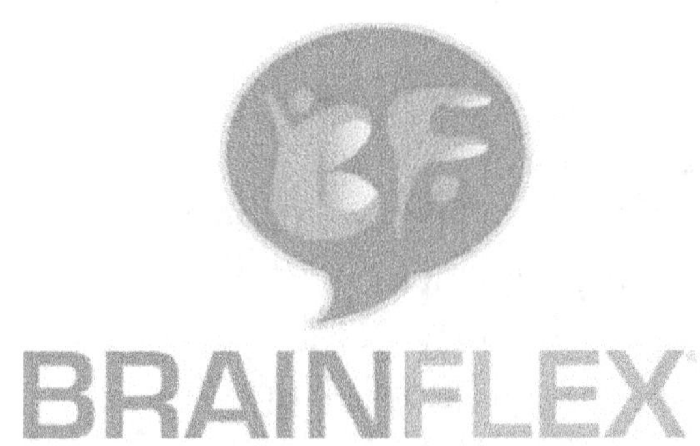

LESSON 1
ANSWERS

PG 1 - Answers to Lesson 1

Answers to Brainagrams

1. Ice Man
2. Admirer
3. Races
4. Taps
5. Eat

6. Costar
7. Evil
8. Angel
9. Hare
10. Generate

Answers to Associated Words - Language Center

1. Done for you
2. Heavy - Rain - Check - Book - Keeper
3. Pain - Killer - Bee - Line - Drive
4. Table - Lamp - Shade - Tree - Branch
5. Feeling - Blue - Sky - Light - Switch
6. Men's - Suit - Case - Study - Hall
7. Cold - Shoulder - Bag - Lady - Bug
8. Come - Back - Door - Stop - Sign

Answers to Trivia: 'LOVE'

1. b. A Kiss and a Hug
2. b. Eros
3. a. Venus
4. a. His own Psyche
5. a. Dom Perignon
6. b. 1901
7. b. Juno
8. b. A Signature Rose 9.
a. Vinegar
10. b. Prison
11. b. The Duke of Orleans
12. a. 1415 (1400's)
13. c. 50 Million
14. a. Richard Cadbury
15. c. 220,000

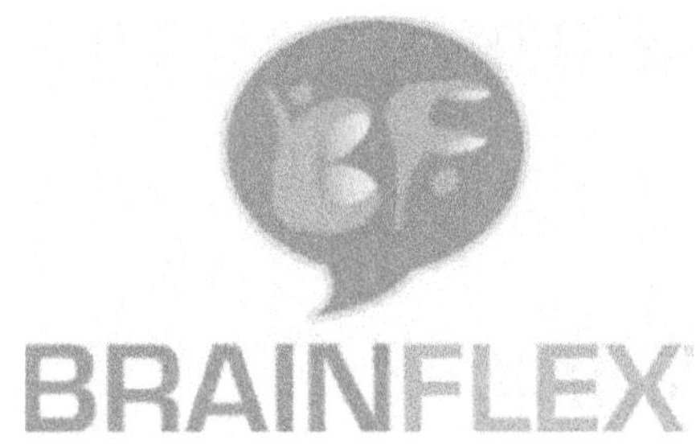

Lesson
2

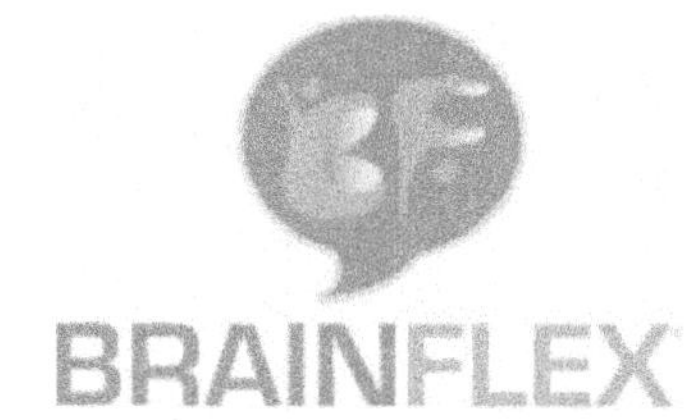

Reminder Page

Don't forget to check off the following after you complete them today:

_____ **Exercise**

_____ **Prayer/Meditation**

_____ **Self-Affirmations**

Self-Affirmations

I have a strong body and a healthy brain.

I free myself of all bitterness and unforgiveness.

I can see my true beauty…within and without.

I choose to assume and believe the best about others.

I choose to believe what God says about me.

I am loved and accepted by those I love.

<u>L</u>ESSON 2: RESEARCH & DISCUSSION
News you can use, and share with others too!

MEMORY STORAGE

Many believe our memories are stored in our brains like books are on a shelf. However, the truth is…our memories are stored in various areas of the brain through a complicated encoding process. In other words, there may be portions of the same memory located in many areas of the brain.

1) We can experience the challenge of retrieving a memory at any time, however there are also times when this is more of a challenge because of an impairment to the brain by a disease or an event that caused injury to the brain.

   a) What can we do to strengthen our memory and recall?

      i) Participate in activities that strengthen neural pathways.

      ii) Find ways to retrieve memories through engaging areas of the brain that retain information the longest, such as those areas in which music and rhythm are stored.

      iii) Be intentional about paying close attention if there is something we want to be certain to remember.

         1) If we aren't paying attention during the time a memory is created, it will be more difficult to recall it later. (Writing information down is very helpful.)

      iv) We may often have a difficult time recalling a memory because it wasn't processed appropriately.

         1) When this occurs, the memory may come to us during a time when we aren't actually trying to recall it. This can happen when something we aren't even aware of triggers the memory.

         (Triggers can be a great tool to assist with recall!)

References

Memory Storage. (2018, February 21). Retrieved from The Human Brain: http://www.human-memory.net/processes_storage.html

Exercise: Circuit Training for the Brain. (P-1)
Recall and Creativity

Read the story below, then give your creative skills a good workout by following the directions on the next page. When you're finished, you'll have the opportunity to exercise your recall.

This Saturday, Gwen and Gary will have been dating for one year. To celebrate, Gary wants to take Gwen to an expensive restaurant in the heart of downtown Boston. However, when he approached Gwen with the idea, she told him that she'd prefer to stay home and watch football that night. Gwen continued with the plans she had already laid out in her mind. "I could order some pizza, and have it delivered right to the house!" she said with excitement. What Gwen doesn't know is that Gary is planning on asking her to marry him, which is why he wanted to make the night so special. What Gary doesn't know is that Gwen has no desire to get married, too anyone, ever.

As Saturday approached, they agreed to stay in and watch football. Even though they weren't going out, Gary had still thought of a creative way to propose. Gwen decided to go ahead and order dinner. She called her favorite pizza place and ordered a medium supreme, which was $13.75. To surprise Gary, she added his favorite appetizer, buffalo wings, to the order, which brought the total up to $27.55. After hanging up, she realized there wasn't a single drink in her fridge, so she quickly called Pizza Ranch back and asked them to add a 2-liter of sugar free iced tea to her order, which brought the total to $30.62.

During halftime, Gary suggested they go sit on Gwen's balcony to get some fresh air. They both settled into the antique Adirondack chairs, when Gwen suddenly noticed a large group of people walking into her yard, and it looked like each person was carrying two candles, one in each hand. She gasped and looked at Gary, with eyes wide opened and said, "Ummm, Gary, what is this?"

Gary got down on one knee and said,

"Gwen, I have gathered 15 of our friends and family together to witness this important day." If you stand up and look over the balcony,you'll be able to see that the candles they're holding form a question, which is the most important question I'll ever ask.

(Now, it's up to you to finish the story on the following page.)

<u>**Exercise: Circuit Training for the Brain (P-2)**</u> Exercise your creative sk ills, (using creative liberty), and finish the story:

____

____

____

____

____

Do your best to answer the following questions without looking back at the story, however if you need to peek, that's okay too. ☺

1. Exercise your math skills by answering the following:
a. What was the cost of the appetizer Gwen ordered for Gary? $________
b. What was the cost of the ice-tea Gwen added to theorder? c. Gwen gave the delivery driver a 20% tip, which was…(?) $________

2. Exercise your short-term memory by answering the following:
(Do your best not to look back at the story.)

   a. Gary wanted to take Gwen to a nice restaurant in the city. In what city was the restaurant located? ________________

   b. Gwen decided to surprise Gary with his favorite appetizer, which was (?) ________________ ________________

   c. What was the name of the restaurant Gwen called to place her order? ________________ ________________

   d. During which part of the game did Gary take Gwen out to the balcony? ________________

   e. While on the back porch, Gwen and Gary sat in what type of chairs? ________________________________

3. Exercise your math skills one more time by determining how many candles were held by Gwen & Gary's friends as they walked into the back yard. ____________

4. Use your creative liberty once again to *imagine* the 'why' behind Gwen's resistance to marriage. ________________________________

____

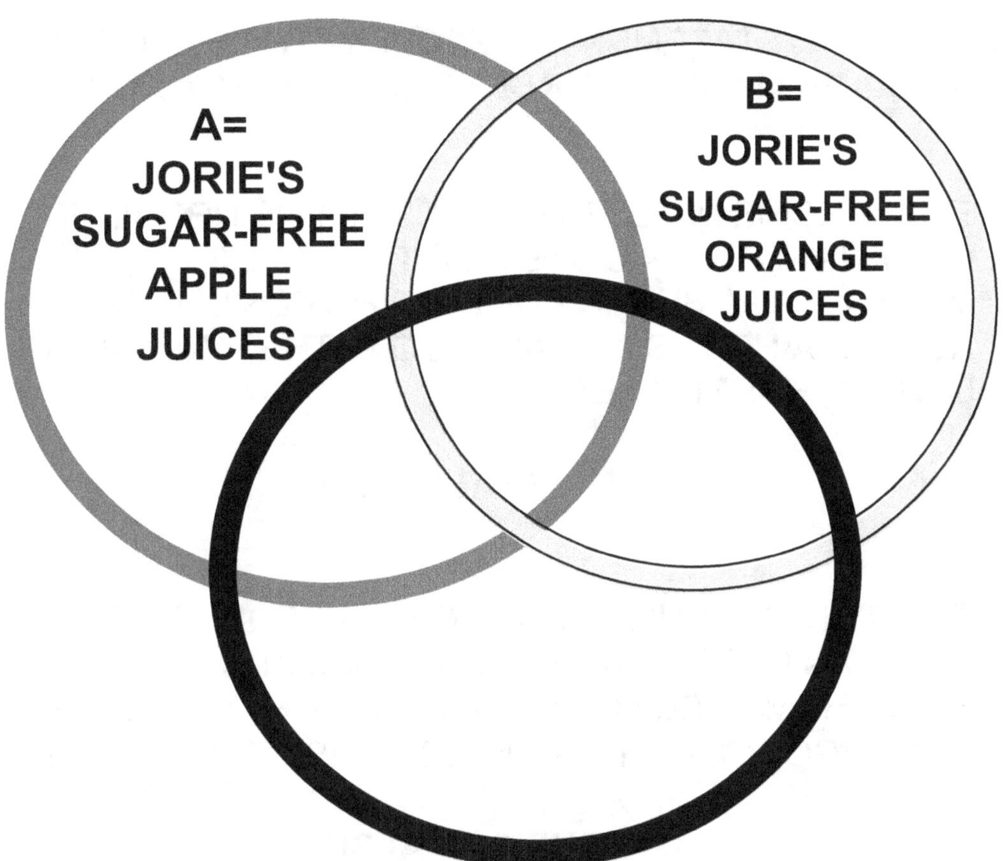

**REVIEW THE STATEMENT BELOW ALONG WITH
THE VENN DIAGRAM ABOVE, THEN CIRCLE THE
THE CORRECT ANSWER.**

IF ALL APPLE JUICE MADE BY JORIE IS SUGAR
FREE (A), AND ALL ORANGE JUICE MADE BY
JORIE (B) IS SUGAR FREE, THEN ALL GRAPE
JUICE MADE BY JORIE IS SUGAR FREE (C)

TRUE or FALSE

NEXT, PLACE THE LETTER **'C'**,
(WHICH REPRESENTS ALL GRAPE JUICE MADE BY JORIE),
IN THE CORRECT LOCATION ON THE VENN DIAGRAM.

1. REVIEW THE STATEMENTS BELOW, WITHOUT THE USE OF A VENN DIAGRAM, THEN CIRCLE THE CORRECT ANSWER.

A. EVERY HOME IN FLORIDA SINCE 1985 IS REQUIRED TO WITHSTAND HURRICANES, UP TO LEVEL 3.
IN 1998, MAGA BEGAN BUILDING HOMES IN FLORIDA.
ALL MAGA HOMES ARE ABLE TO WITHSTAND, UP TO LEVEL 3, HURRICANES.

TRUE OR FALSE

B. EVERY HOME BUILT IN FLORIDA IS REQUIRED TO PASS AN EXTENSIVE SAFETY INSPECTION.
LAGO HOMES BUILDS HOMES IN FLORIDA AND GEORGIA.
ALL LAGO HOMES PASS AN EXTENSIVE SAFETY TEST.

TRUE OR FALSE

C. ALL ORANGE TREES GROW IN A WARM CLIMATE.
MISSISSIPPI IS A WARM CLIMATE.
ALL ORANGE TREES GROW IN MISSISSIPPI.

TRUE OR FALSE

D. ACCORDING TO THE FOUNDING DOCUMENTS OF THE USA, CERTAIN HUMAN RIGHTS ARE GIVEN BY GOD AND CANNOT BE TAKEN AWAY. FREEDOM OF SPEECH AND FREEDOM OF RELIGION ARE RIGHTS GIVEN FROM GOD. FREEDOM OF SPEECH AND FREEDOM OF RELIGION CANNOT BE TAKEN AWAY.

TRUE OR FALSE

LONG-TERM MEMORY CHALLENGE
TRIVIA: Christmas Any Time of Year

1. In what year was the first 'Rockefeller Center Christmas Tree'
   put up on display?
   - a. 1933
   - b. 1953
   - c. 1963

2. As of 2021, what Northeastern US state held the Guinness record for the
   largest snowman?
   - a. Maryland
   - b. Maine
   - c. Pennsylvania

3. As of the year 2021, how tall was the tallest cut Christmas tree?
   - a. appx. 20 feet
   - b. appx. 100 feet
   - c. appx. 200 feet

4. Who created the first electric light Christmas display?
   - a.Thomas Edison
   - b. Dwight Eisenhower
   - c. Amadeus Mozart

5. To what country is the Poinsettia, with its red and green leaves,
   native?
   - a. Austria
   - b. Mexico
   - c. Canada

6. What large former retail outlet commissioned and published
   'Rudolph the Re-Nosed Reindeer"?
   - a. Macy's
   - b. Montgomery Ward
   - c. Woolworth's

7. How many wise men/Magi/kings, does the Bible say visited the baby Jesus?
    a. 3
    b. 7
    c. It doesn't say

8. Up until the year 2021, what was the most popular meal for many Japanese families on Christmas Day?
    a. Pheasant
    b. Rum & Noodles
    c. KFC Fried Chicken

9. What Southeast Asian Country has the longest holiday season, which starts in September and continues through January?
    a. The Philippines
    b. South Korea
    c. None of the Above

10. This cartoon character may be seen hanging out with Mickey Mouse.
    a. Donald Duck
    b. Bugs Bunny
    c. Scooby Doo

11. In which country did the Christmas tree originate?
    a. China
    b. The United States
    c. Germany

12. What 'plant based' tradition requires an expression of love when one find's themselves standing under it with someone of the opposite sex?
    a. Pulling buttons from pudding made of plums
    b. A hanging mistletoe
    c. Finding a pickle hidden in the Christmas tree

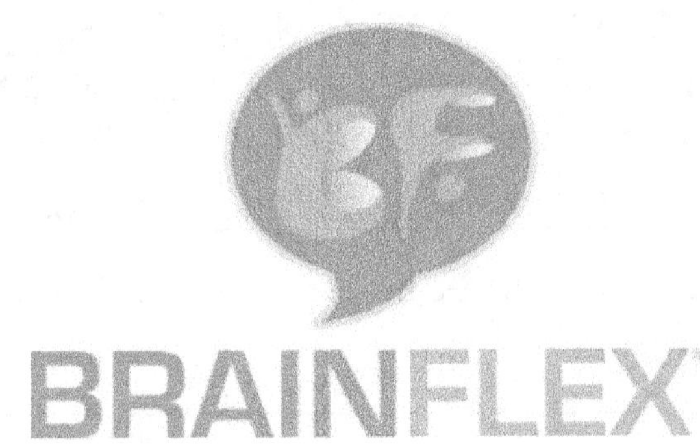

LESSON 2
ANSWERS

Answers to Lesson 2

Answers to 'Exercise Circuit Training for the Brain'

1. a. How much was the appetizer Gwen ordered for Gary? **$13.80**
   The pizza was $13.75, after she ordered the appetizer the total order was $27.56. ($27.55 - $13.75 = **$13.80**)
   b. How much was the ice-tea Gwen added to the order? **$3.07**
   The order was up to $27.55. After the tea was added, the order was $30.62. ($30.62 - $27.55 = **$3.07**)
   c. Gwen gave the delivery driver a 20% tip, which was..?) **$6.12**
   The total order was $30.62. (10% is $3.06 x 2 = **$6.12**)

2. [a] **Boston** [b] **Buffalo Wings** [c] **Pizza Ranch** [d] **Half-Time** [e] **Adirondack**

3. 15 friends had a candle in each hand. 15 x 2 = **30 candles**
4. **Will You Marry Me**

With the information we have been given, we can conclude the following:

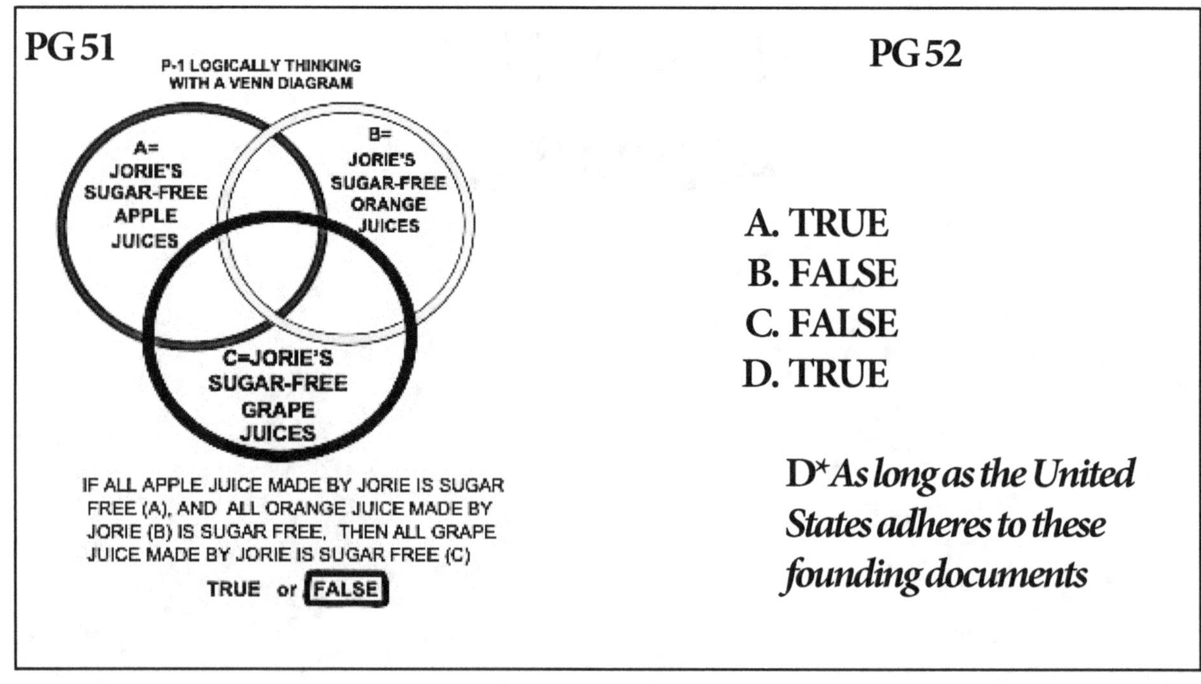

ANSWERS TO LESSON 2

ANSWERS: LONG-TERM MEMORY CHALLENGE TRIVIA: Christmas Any Time of Year

1. What was the first year the Rockefeller Center Christmas Tree was put up on display?
    a. **<u>1933</u>**
    b. 1953
    c. 1963

2. What Northeastern US state holds the Guinness record for the largest snowman?
    a. Maryland
    b. **<u>Maine</u>**
    c. Pennsylvania

3. How tall was the tallest cut Christmas tree?
    a. appx. 20 feet
    b. appx. 100 feet
    c. **<u>appx. 200 feet</u>**

4. Who created the first electric light Christmas display?
    a. **<u>Thomas Edison</u>**
    b. Dwight Eisenhower
    c. Amadeus Mozart

5. In what country is the Poinsettia, with its red and green leaves, native to?
    a. Austria
    b. **<u>Mexico</u>**
    c. Canada

6. What large former retail outlet commissioned and published 'Rudolph the Red nosed Reindeer'?
    a. Macy's
    b. **<u>Montgomery Ward</u>**
    c. Woolworth's

ANSWERS TO: LONG-TERM MEMORY CHALLENGE TRIVIA:
Christmas Any Time of Year

7. How many wise men/Magi/kings, does the Bible say visited the baby Jesus?
    a. 3
    b. 7
    c. **It doesn't say**

8. What is the most popular meal for Christmas in Japan?
    a. Pheasant
    b. Rum & Noodles
    c. **KFC Fried Chicken**

9. What Southeast Asian Country has the longest holiday season, which starts in September and continues through January?
    a. **The Philippines**
    b. South Korea
    c. None of the Above

10. Which cartoon character is a Christmas Eve tradition in Sweden and is watched by millions of Swedes every year?
    a. **Donald Duck**
    b. Bugs Bunny
    c. Mickey Mouse

11. In which country did the Christmas tree originate?
    a. China
    b. The United States
    c. **Germany**

12. What 'plant based' tradition requires an expression of love when one find's themselves standing under it with someone of the opposite sex?
    a. Pulling buttons from pudding made of plums
    b. **A hanging mistletoe**
    c. Finding a pickle hidden in the Christmas tree

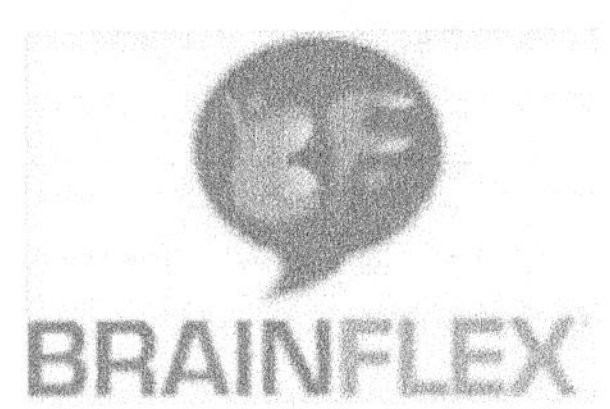

Week Two
NUTRITIONAL RECIPE

Contributing to a healthier brain & body

The health benefits in the recipe's ingredients will vary with each individual and depend heavily upon each person's level of commitment to making healthy life-style choices on a consistent basis.

Bruschetta Chicken over Spinach

INGREDIENTS-Serves 1

¼ cup **pre-cooked** grilled chicken breast-diced
(Allow time to thaw) (Can be purchased in the freezer section)

¼ cup fresh organic spinach leaves

2 Tbsp bruschetta *(tomato, basil, onion, garlic, salt/pepper)*
(Can be purchased already made fresh in the deli)

1 Tbsp shredded mozzarella or parmesan cheese
(not processed)

Balsamic Vinaigrette to drizzle as a dressing

Instructions

1.) Allow pre-cooked frozen chicken breast to thaw

2.) If you prefer to have your chicken warm, you can place it in the microwave for 45 seconds. *(Note: Microwaving food is not the best practice if you want to be sure your food maintains its nutrients.)*

3.) Place spinach leaves on plate, then top w/chicken

4.) Spread bruschetta over top of chicken & spinach

5.) Drizzle balsamic vinaigrette dressing

6.) Sprinkle shredded cheese on top

Health Benefits: Tomatoes

- **Full of antioxidants, which the immune system needs to help our body fight against disease**

  - **These antioxidants also equip our body to battle cancer causing free radicals, which is why tomatoes are said to help decrease the risk of many types of cancer.**

- **Nutrients in tomatoes help supports cardiovascular health.**

- **Folic acid in tomatoes has been shown to help battle depression.**

Health Benefits: Onions

Considered to be 'Nutrient Dense', which means
they are low in calories & high in vitamins & minerals.

Have been shown to contribute to heart health.

Full of antioxidants, which support the immune system
and fight cancer causing free radicals in our system.

Helps control blood sugar levels & increase bone density.

Has antibacterial properties, battling against the bad
bacteria in the body.

Beneficial to our digestive health.

Health Benefits: Spinach

-Spinach has been shown to lower the risk of complications
associated with diabetes.

-The Vitamin A in spinach contributes to eye health.

-Contains antioxidants that boost the immune system.

-The calcium in spinach supports bone strength.

This is especially important, since bone density decreases w/age.

-Spinach has been shown to lower the protein levels that
contribute to heart disease.

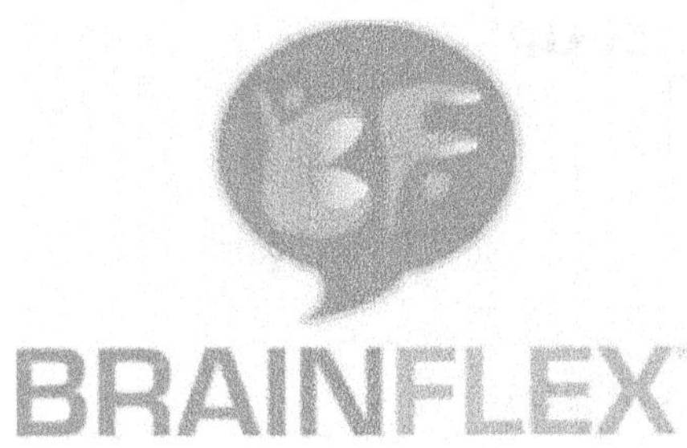

BRAINFLEX

Lesson
3

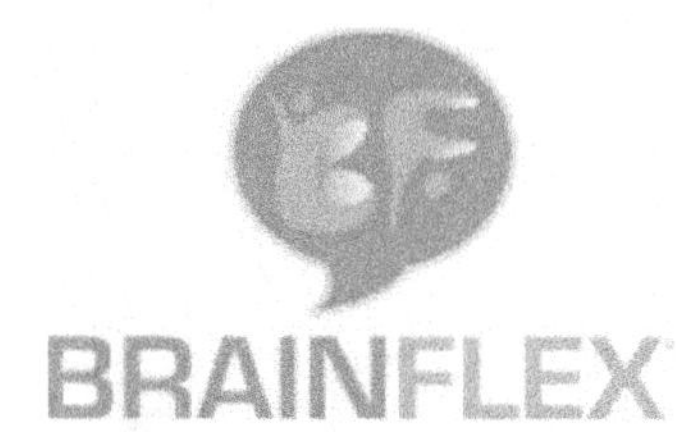

<u>Reminder Page</u>

Don't forget to check off the following after you complete them today:

_____ **Exercise**

_____ **Prayer/Meditation**

_____ **Self-Affirmations**

SELF AFFIRMATIONS

I AM CAPABLE AND STRONG.

MY CONFIDENCE IS INCREASING.

GOD WILL STRENGTHEN ME TO DO THE THINGS I NEED TO DO.

I AM PROTECTED FROM THE NEGATIVE WORDS OF OTHERS.

NO ONE DECIDES MY VALUE AND WORTH.

LESSON 3: RESEARCH & DISCUSSION

News you can use, (and share with others too.)

Brain-Nutrition Connection

The 'MIND' diet, (similar to the 'Mediterranean Diet') along with foods found in 'The Blue Zones', is considered by many research scientists to be 'neuro-protective'. (It is from these guidelines that we create some of our BrainFlex recipes.) Many of the foods included in these particular recipes have been shown to help prevent Alzheimer's and other diseases that cause or contribute to dementia. A few examples of these types of foods are salmon, avocado, spinach, tomatoes, blue berries, and almonds. For decades, we have been aware of the impact that food has on our health. We know that a diet high in the wrong types of fat and carbs can break down in the body. This can result in high blood pressure/hypertension, heart disease, or type 2 diabetes. Numerous studies have shown that what we eat also impacts our brain health. It is now understood that the right nutrition has a positive impact on brain health and can deter or slow down memory loss.

In addition, since high blood pressure, type 2 diabetes, and cardiovascular disease are now considered to be contributors to 'Alzheimer's disease', we can safely say that healthy eating plays a large role in the prevention or slowing down of cognitive decline. The stomach is considered to be the 'second brain' and there is a direct connection between the two. Dr. Caroline Leaf, a Cognitive Neuroscientist, stated the following, "Our thought life impacts our digestive system, and our digestive system impacts our brain." Her research confirms that our mind effects our stomach and what we put in our stomach effects our minds, and because of this, we know that what we eat heavily influences our entire well-being.

Works Cited
Elise Mandi, B. (2018, January 28). healthline.com. Retrieved from The Worst Foods for Your
      Brain: https://www.healthline.com/nutrition/worst-foods-for-your-brain

Challenge your long-term memory by answering the following questions, but keep in mind, the rule of Jeopardy is that you must answer each question with a question. Some of the challenges below are simple words we rarely use, others may be a bit more difficult.

1. She jumped down a rabbit hole and found herself in a new and amazing place. **Who is?** _______________________________

2. In this movie, Holly Golightly both shines like a diamond in the morning and cries like a lost and lonely cat stuck in the evening rain. **What is** _______________________________

3. After being hit on the head with an apple, this man discovered gravity. **Who is** _______________________________

4. This president and 'alleged' tree chopper may have never eaten cherry pie. **Who is** _______________________________

5. This begins with ice and buttermilk, then a few extra sugary items are added to make a delicious dessert, which can bring great enjoyment, especially when chocolate fudge is added.
What is _______________________

6. She wanted terribly to be involved in her husband's 'show biz' world, but her sneaky attempts, sometimes involving her best friend Ethel, were all to no avail.
Who is _______________________________

7. This mixture, once water is added, is applied between bricks to help create the structure of a building.
What is _______________________________

8. This branch of the government includes the supreme court.
What is _______________________________

9. This man was loved in Hollywood and in the 1980's, he was loved in Washington D.C., when he served as the 40th President of the United States. **Who is** _______________________

10. Born as 'Norma Jeane Mortenson, her name was changed shortly after becoming America's blond bomb shell; but sadly, she passed away at age 36. **Who is** _______________________________

11. This country hosts the cities of Vancouver and Toronto.
    What is _______________________

12. This ocean borders the east side of the United States.
    What is _______________________________________

13. Plug its cord into the wall and use to make cutting turkey and ham a bit easier. **What is** _______________________________

14. This song is about a brightly colored aquatic vessel, where 'we all lived'. **What is** _______________________________

15. This man became President of the United States after Nixon resigned, and shares the same last name with one of America's greatest inventors. **Who is** _____________________________

16. This 1970's country television show starred Buck Owens, Roy Clarke and Grandpa Jones, and featured a song w/the lyrics, "If it weren't for bad luck, I'd have no luck at all."
    What is _______________________________________

17. This actor was well known for his many talents, which included both singing and acting, however, he is often best remembered from his television show, which highlighted his turbulent relation-with 'Sargent Carter' in the Navy.
    Who is _____________________________

18. This city, located in Missouri, hosts the large "Arch", which represents the 'Gateway to the West'.
    What is _____________________________

19. Raindrops on roses, whiskers on kittens, bright copper kettles and warm woolen mittens might be listed in this well-known song.
    What are _______________________________________

20. This little red-headed girl with braids, represents one of the best hamburgers around, (and will serve you a chocolate 'Frosty' too.)
    Who is _____________________________

Exercise: Solving Word Problems ~ Thought Process

Read the paragraph below, then answer the questions that follow.

Jonathan just landed a new accounting job at the 'Flex Club' in the heart of downtown Columbus, Ohio. He has leased a condo 2 miles from his new office. Physical fitness is very important to Jonathan, so he's decided to either walk or ride his bike to work. He figured out that it will take him 20 minutes to ride his bike to work and 40 minutes to walk.

1. How many minutes will it take Jonathan to walk 1/2 of a mile? _________

2. On his first day of work, Jonathan road his bike. He left his house at 7:30 am. What time did Jonathan get to work that morning? __________

3. The next day, Jonathan walked to work. That morning, one of his new friends invited to lunch at 'Mama D's, a local Italian restaurant, which required a 20-minute walk from the office, in the opposite direction of his home. When Jonathan finally arrived home that evening, how many extra mile(s) had he walked that day? _________ How many total minutes had he walked that day?________   Convert this to hours. _______

4. Monday morning Jonathan decided that he should do a better job planning his week. So he grabbed a pad of paper and began writing down his plan. He would walk to work every Monday, Wednesday, and Friday, and ride his bike every Tuesday and Thursday.
   a. Total the amount of time, in minutes, that Jonathan will spend riding his bike each week, in minutes. __________
   b. Total the amount of time he will spend walking to work each week, in minutes. ______
   c. Calculate the total amount of time Jonathan will spend commuting to work each week, in minutes.________
      Convert to hours (and minutes) _________

5. Jonathan was excited for his grandparents to see his new condo, so he invited them to visit. They live in Cincinnati, Ohio, which is about 150 miles from Jonathan's home. If they set their cruise control at 60 MPH, approximately how long will it take them to get to their grandson's condo? ________ hours and __________ minutes.

Part 1 Exercise: Long-term memory with Spatial Orientation

First, cover the bottom section of this page. Next, fill in the names of *at least* 30 states, doing your best not to look at the answers below.

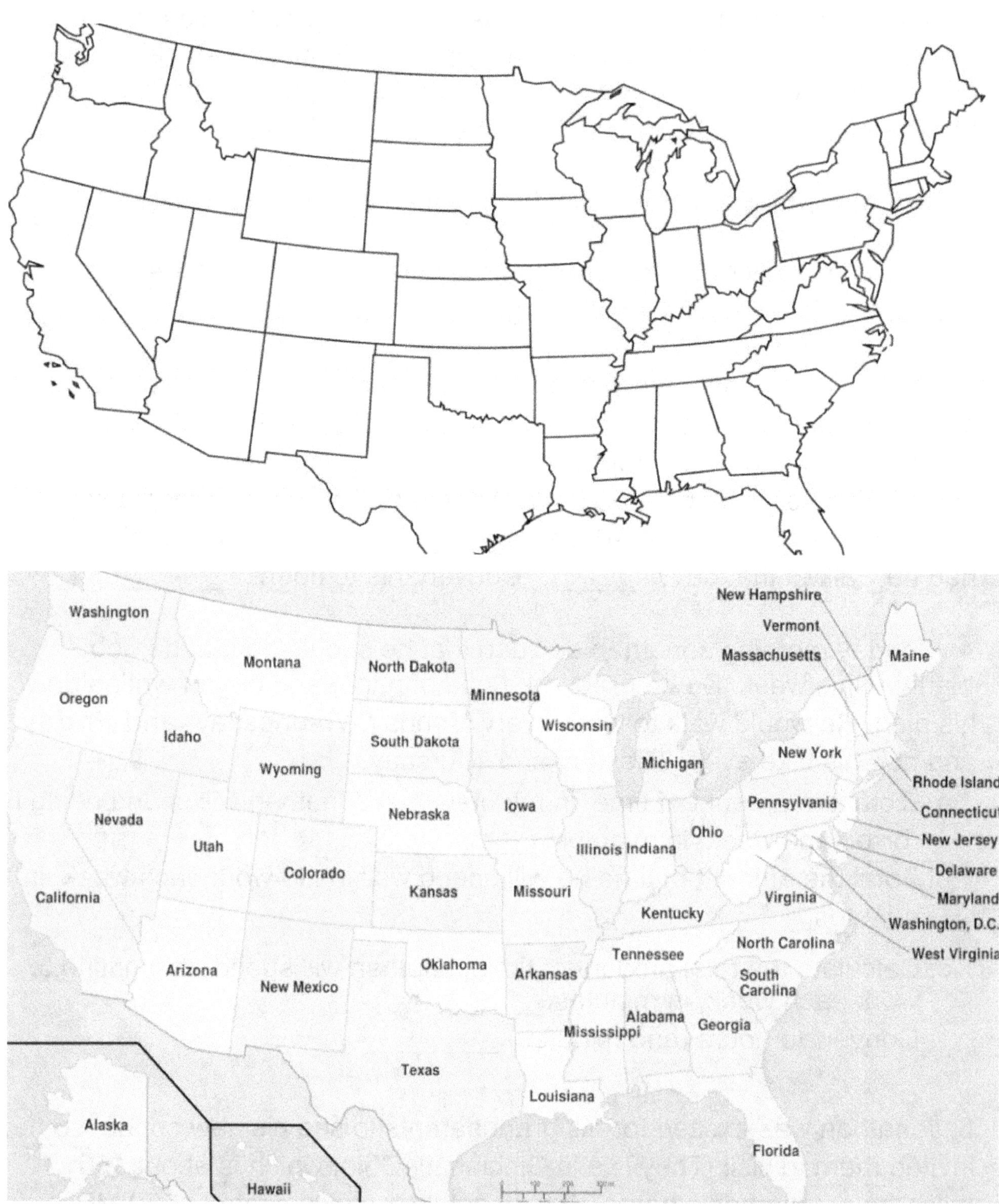

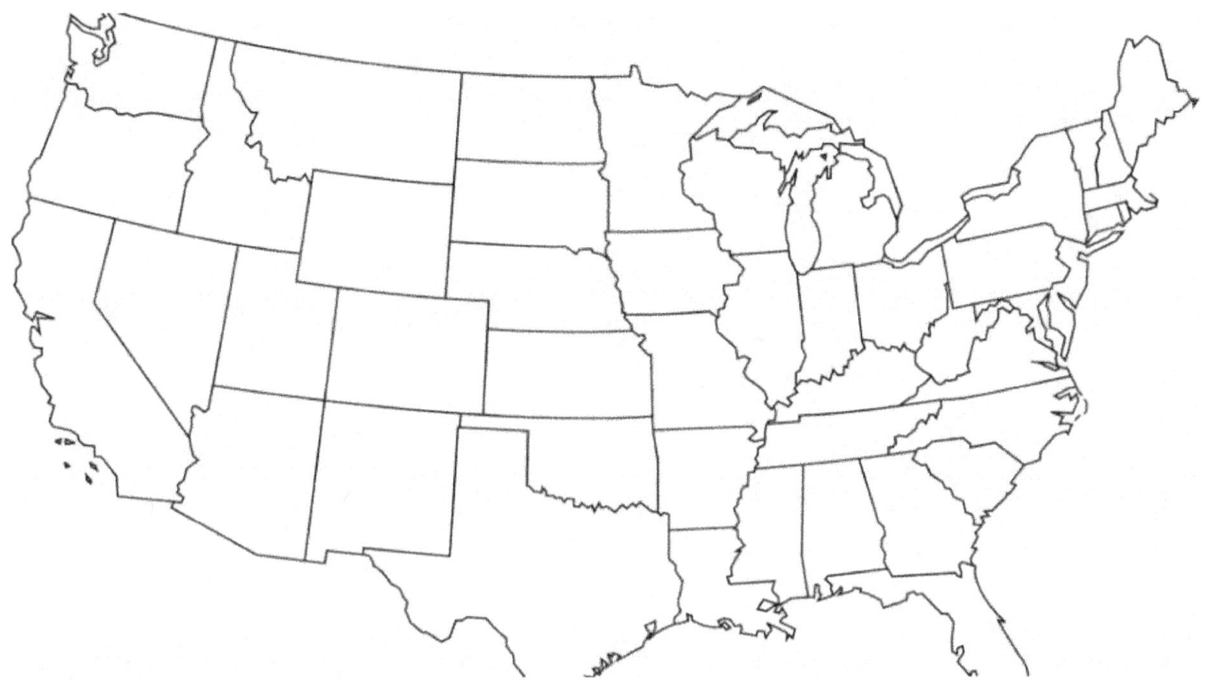

Abbreviation	Capital	State	Abbreviation	Capital	State
AL	MONTGOMERY	ALABAMA	MT	HELENA	MONTANA
AK	JUNEAU	ALASKA	NE	LINCOLN	NEBRASKA
AZ	PHOENIX	ARIZONA	NV	CARSON CITY	NEVADA
AR	LITTLE ROCK	ARKANSAS	NH	CONCORD	NEW HAMPSHIRE
CA	SACRAMENTO	CALIFORNIA	NJ	TRENTON	NEW JERSEY
CO	DENVER	COLORADO	NM	SANTA FE	NEW MEXICO
CT	HARTFORD	CONNECTICUT	NY	ALBANY	NEW YORK
DE	DOVER	DELAWARE	NC	RALEIGH	NORTH CAROLINA
FL	TALLAHASSEE	FLORIDA	ND	BISMARCK	NORTH DAKOTA
GA	ATLANTA	GEORGIA	OH	COLUMBUS	OHIO
HI	HONOLULU	HAWAII	OK	OKLAHOMA CITY	OKLAHOMA
ID	BOISE	IDAHO	OR	SALEM	OREGON
IL	SPRINGFIELD	ILLINOIS	PA	HARRISBURG	PENNSYLVANIA
IN	INDIANAPOLIS	INDIANA	RI	PROVIDENCE	RHODE ISLAND
IA	DES MOINES	IOWA	SC	COLUMBIA	SOUTH CAROLINA
KS	TOPEKA	KANSAS	SD	PIERRE	SOUTH DAKOTA
KY	FRANKFORT	KENTUCKY	TN	NASHVILLE	TENNESSEE
LA	BATON ROUGE	LOUISIANA	TX	AUSTIN	TEXAS
ME	AUGUSTA	MAINE	UT	SALT LAKE CITY	UTAH
MD	ANNAPOLIS	MARYLAND	VT	MONTPELIER	VERMONT
MA	BOSTON	MASSACHUSETTS	VA	RICHMOND	VIRGINIA
MI	LANSING	MICHIGAN	WA	OLYMPIA	WASHINGTON
MN	ST. PAUL	MINNESOTA	WV	CHARLESTON	WEST VIRGINIA
MS	JACKSON	MISSISSIPPI	WI	MADISON	WISCONSIN
MO	JEFFERSON CITY	MISSOURI	WY	CHEYENNE	WYOMING

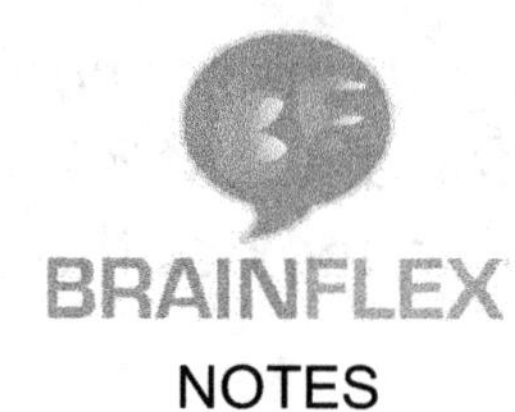

BRAINFLEX
NOTES

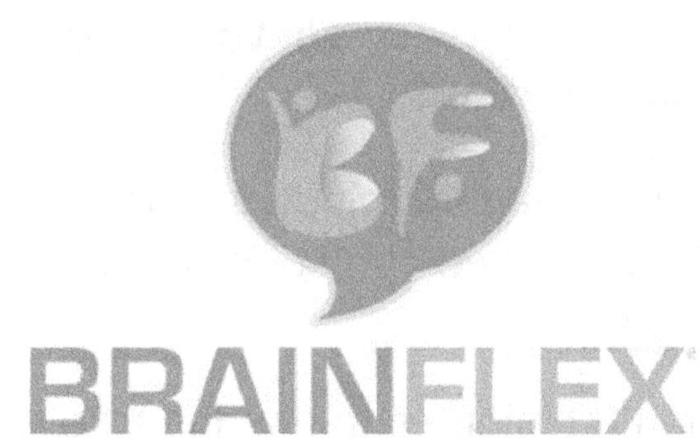

LESSON 3
ANSWERS

Answers to BrainFlex Jeopardy

1. Who is Alice in Wonderland?
2. What is Breakfast at Tiffany's?
3. Who is Sir Isaac Newton?
4. Who is George Washington?
5. What is Ice Cream?
6. Who is Lucille Ball?
7. What is Mortar?
8. What is the Judicial Branch?
9. Who is Ronald Reagan?
10. Who is Marilyn Monroe?
11. What is Canada?
12. What is the Atlantic Ocean?
13. What is an Electric Knife?
14. What is the Yellow Submarine?
15. Who is Gerald Ford?
16. What is 'Hee Haw'?
17. Who is Gomer Pyle? Or Jim Neighbors
18. What is the St. Louis?
19. What are a few of my favorite things?
20. Who is Wendy?

Answers to Exercise: Solving Word Problems ~ Thought Process

1. **10 minutes** If it takes Jonathan 40 minutes to walk 2 miles, it would take him 20 minutes to walk 1 mile, so we can conclude that it would take him **10 minutes to walk ½ of a mile.**

2. **7:50** If it takes Jonathan 20 minutes to ride his bike to work and he left his home at 7:30, then **his arrival time would be 7:50.**

3. **2 miles** The restaurant was a 40 minute walk, round trip. It takes Jonathan 40 minutes to walk 2 miles.
120 minutes   It takes Jonathan 80 minutes to walk to and from work, and he walked an extra 40 minutes to walk to the restaurant. 80+40=120 min.
2 hours (60 minutes in one hour, 120 minutes - 2 hrs.)

4. **160 min.** Jonathan plans to walk 2 days/wk. 40min x 2=80 x 2(RT) =160
120 min. Jonathan plans to ride his bike 3 days/wk. 20min x 3 = 60x2(RT) =120
4 hours and 40 minutes (60 minutes in 1 hour: 280 min.= 4 hrs. and 40 min.)

5. **2 hours and 30 minutes** If Jonathan's grandparents drive 60 miles an hour and they live 150 miles away, it will take them 2 and ½ hours to get to Jonathan's home.

One way to solve this math problem is to consider that there are 60 minutes in an hour, so if they drive 60 miles every hour, they are driving 1 mile every minute, which is 150 minutes. When this is converted to hours/minutes, it is **2 hours and 30 minutes**

Answers to Map Challenges are within the activity.

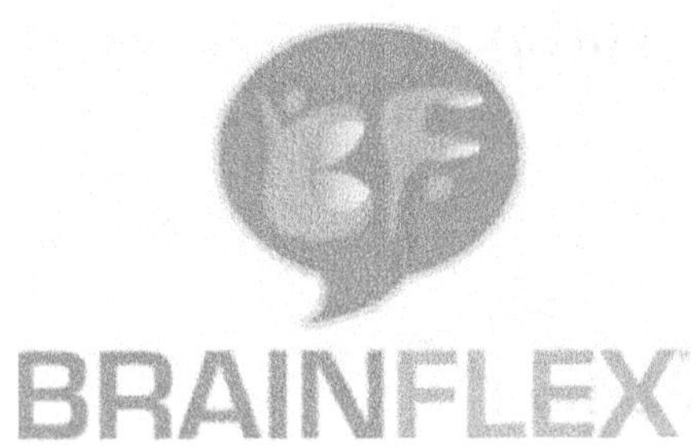

Lesson
4

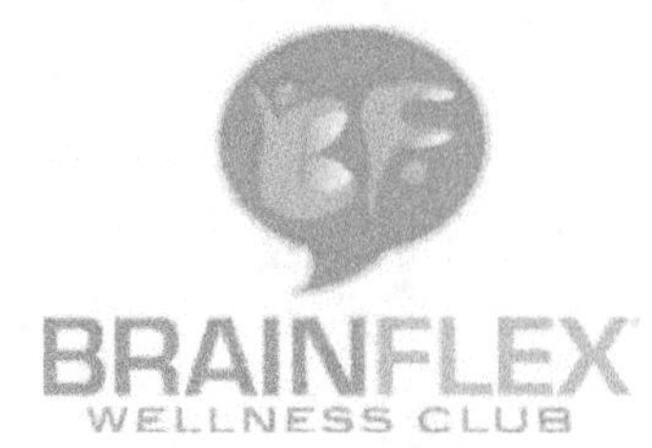

Reminder Page

Don't forget to check off the following after you complete them today:

_____ Exercise

_____ Prayer/Meditation

_____ Self-Affirmations

<u>SELF-AFFIRMATIONS</u>

What I do does not determine my worth.

I am worthy of love and respect.

I love myself and others.

I am loved by those who are important to me.

I am safe and protected by God.

I refuse to allow my mind to worry.

I am grateful for the life I have been given.

<u>**Lesson 4: Research & Discussion**</u>
Exercising Various Types of Thinking Skills
(News you can use and share with others too!)

If you walked into the kitchen and saw a watermelon inside a milk jug, sealed tightly with no sign of tampering, what would you think? You would likely find yourself scratching your head while trying to figure out just how this could have happened. Situations like this require both logical and illogical (out of the box) thinking, and you'll probably need to call on your critical thinking skills as well.

Of course, you aren't likely to ever be in this situation; however, figuring out these types of scenarios can help keep your mind sharp and strengthen your ability to solve other problems. If we take the time to stop and think about it, we'll quickly realize that we make decisions all day, every day…throughout the entire year. What should I have for breakfast? Should I believe what I just heard on the news? Do I need to wear a jacket to the store? Should I move my money to another investment? How much should I spend on a new car? How much should I budget for Christmas?

In addition to decisions, there are also debates we'd like to win. However, this requires us to reason, think outside of box and engage our critical or logical thinking skills. For example, let's say your granddaughter is dating someone and you see signs that concern you and you're convinced he could be trouble. If you want to make a convincing argument, it will require one or more of these types of thinking skills. This is one of many reasons it's so important to keep them sharp.

Quick Overview: What is Critical Thinking?
The best way to understand the difference between critical thinking and other types of thinking is to consider the five w's.
(Who, What, Where, When and Why)
Believe it or not, we quite often engage in critical thinking.
Here are a few simple examples of critical thinking:
1. If I eat too much ice cream, how will I feel? Will I feel bloated and sluggish.
2. If I call to comfort my friend, who is upset about the outcome of the latest election, will it help? Will it change how she is feeling?
3. I have had three fender benders in three months. Why is this happening?
4. Each time I visit a particular friend, I leave feeling depressed? Why?

The following 'Baby Boomer' trivia will give your neural pathways quite a challenge. However, if you aren't sure of the answer, your brain is still benefiting, since new information contributes to the brain's cognitive reserve. The key to learning as we age is repetition and more repetition, so be sure to discuss these trivia questions with others.

1. 'Baby Boomers' were born during what years?

   a. 1938-1950   b. 1940-1960   c. 1946-1964   d. 1949-1969

2. What president made the remark "You won't have President Nixon to kick around anymore?"

   a. Eisenhower   b. Nixon   c. Truman   d. Johnson

3. In what city did the Reverend Dr. Martin Luther King make his famous "I Have A Dream Speech?"

   a. Memphis, TN

   b. Washington D.C.

   c. Selma, AL

   d. Montgomery, AL

4. In 1964, *'The Beatles'* began their first U.S. tour on what show?

   a. The Ed Sullivan Show

   b. Shindig

   c. Hullabaloo

   d. The Steve Allen Show

5. In July of 1966 a group named, 'The Lovin' Spoonful's' topped the charts with which of the following songs?

   a. Daydream

   b. Summer in the City

   c. You Didn't Have to Be So Nice

   d. Do You Believe in Magic?

6. Bill Mazeroski hit a dramatic seventh-game home run, giving the Pittsburgh Pirates a World Series triumph over what team?

    a. Chicago White Sox

    b. New York Yankees

    c. Cleveland Indians

    d. Washington Senators

7. In what year did East Germany begin to erect the Berlin Wall?

    a. 1961   b. 1960   c. 1962   d. 1959

8. What film, (which later became a hit on Broadway), won an Academy Award for '*Best Movie of the Year*' in 1961?

    a. *El Cid*

    b. *Breakfast at Tiffany's*

    c. *West Side Story*

    d. *Two Women*

9. In 1961 Harper Lee won the Pulitzer Prize for '*Best Fiction Book*'. What was the name of this book? (*also became a movie*)

    a. *The Making of a President*

    b. *Guns of Navarone*

    c. *To Kill a Mockingbird*

    d. *Catch-22*

10. This President stirred thousands of college students to join the Peace Corps, which he created.

    a. President John F. Kennedy   b. President Dwight D. Eisenhower

    c. President Harry S. Truman   d. President Lyndon Baines Johnson

<u>Long-Term Memory Working with Creativity</u>

Most of us often look back and think about things we wish we would have done differently or we may wonder if there were times we should have made a different choice. It's safe to say that everyone, at one time or another, has experienced the proverbial 'fork in the road'. Of course, there are some choices that have more impact on our lives than others.

This activity is designed to spark your creative thinking while also engaging your long-term memory. Following are a few questions to get you started:

-Consider the following:
  -What are some of the 'fork in the road' moments you've experienced?
  -Are there certain paths in life you are thankful you decided to take?
  -What would the alternative paths have looked like in these situations?
    -Where would it have taken you?
    -How would your life be different today?

As you ponder these things, write your thoughts below, and then, if you're comfortable doing so, share them with a family member or friend. You can also ask them some of these questions as well. This is a great way to start an interesting conversation, which helps us to connect with others in a special way and can be great advice for the younger generation(s).

____

____

____

____

____

____

____

CHALLENGE: DRAWING WITH NON-DOMINANT HAND
Exercise your brain-hand connection and visual acuity
as you draw each of the items in the adjacent square
using your non-dominant hand.

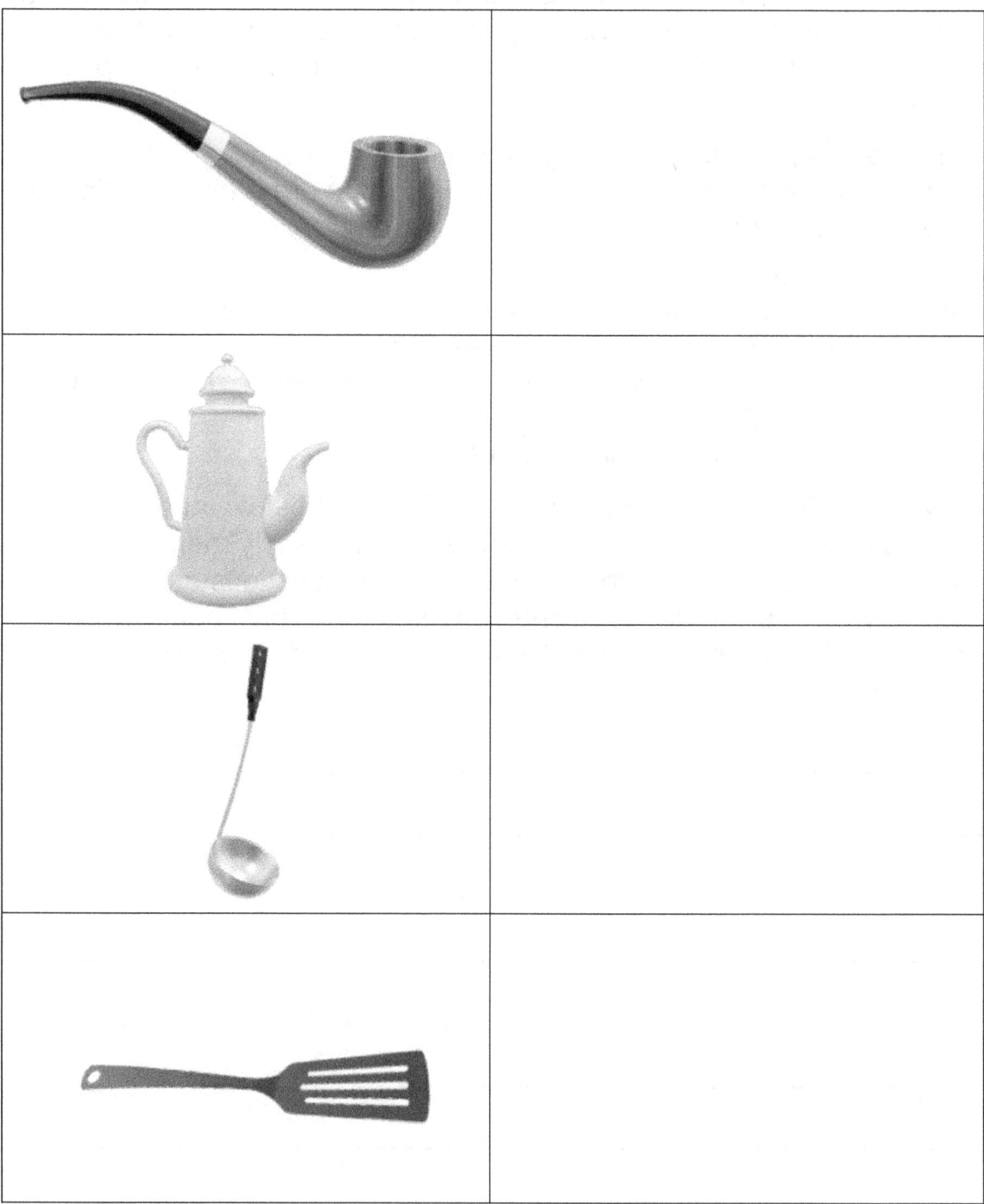

Math Review

Complete the following 'equivalent ratios'. The first one
has been done for you.

First, we determined that 3 was multiplied
by 5 in order to get 15
So, we then multiply 7 by 5 as well (=<u>35</u>)

$3 : 7 = 15 : \underline{35}$

$1 : 4 = 4 : \underline{\hphantom{00}}$

$10 : 3 = \underline{\hphantom{00}} : 6$

$11 : 7 = 22 : \underline{\hphantom{00}}$

$8 : 3 = 32 : \underline{\hphantom{00}}$

$5 : 11 = 20 : \underline{\hphantom{00}}$

$12 : 1 = \underline{\hphantom{00}} : 4$

$1 : 6 = \underline{\hphantom{00}} : 30$

$9 : 4 = 36 : \underline{\hphantom{00}}$

$3 : 5 = \underline{\hphantom{00}} : 20$

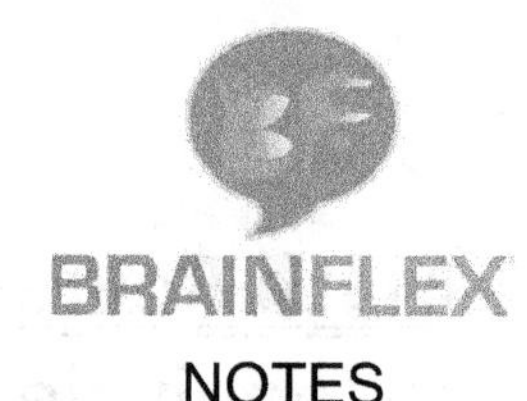

NOTES

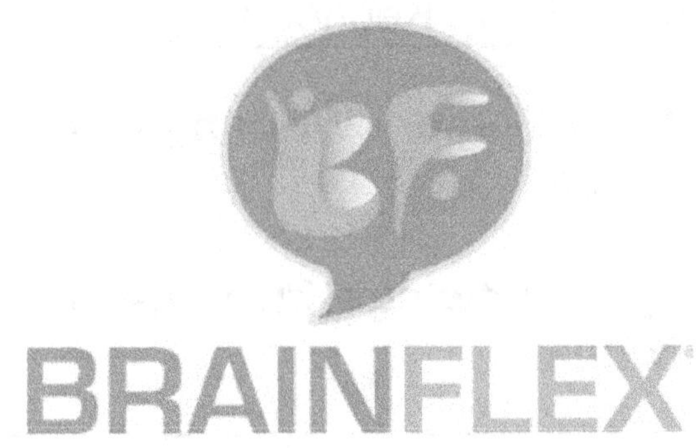

LESSON 4
ANSWERS

Answers to Lesson 4

<u>Answers to Baby Boomer Trivia</u>

1. c. 1946-1964
2. b. President Nixon
3. b. Washington D.C.
4. a. The Ed Sullivan Show
5. b. Summer in the City
6. b. New York Yankees
7. a. 1961
8. c. West Side Story
9. c. To Kill a Mockingbird
10.   a. President John F. Kennedy

Answers to 'Long-Term Memory Working with Creativity' will vary with each individual

Answers to Challenge: 'Drawing with Non-Dominant Hand' will vary with each individual

Answers to Equivalent Ratios

3:7 = 15: **35**
(3x5=15):(7x5=35)

1:4 = 4: **16**
(1x4=4):(4x4=16)

10:3 = 20: **6**
(10x2=20):(3x2=6)

11:7 = 22: **14**
(11x2=22):(7x2=14)

8 : 3 = 32: **12**
(8x4=32):(3x4=12)

5 : 11 = 20 : **44**
(5x4=20):(11x4=44)

12 : 1 = **48** : 4
(1x4=4):(12x4=48)

1 : 6 = **5** : 30
(6x5=30):(1x5=5)

9 : 4 = 36 : **16**
(9x4=36):(4x4=16)

3 : 5 = **12** : 20
(3x4=12):(5x4=20)

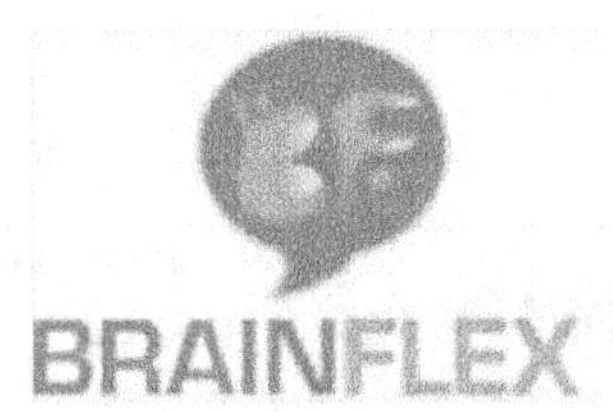

Week Three
NUTRITIONAL RECIPE

Contributing to a
healthier brain & body

The health benefits in the recipe's ingredients will vary with each individual and depend heavily upon each person's level of commitment to making healthy life-style choices on a consistent basis.

| 5 MINUTES TO REFRESHMENT

SALAD DELISH |

INGREDIENTS

- 3-4 cherry tomatoes
- 1 tsp red onions (chopped)
- 1 tsp basil
- tsp garlic salt
- 1/2 cup mozzarella (sliced or chopped)
- 1cup of lettuce (Romaine or Spring Mix)
- 1- 2 tsp of Balsamic Vinaigrette

INSTRUCTIONS

- Wash lettuce and toss into bowl
- Slice/chop mozzarella cheese
- Chop/slice onions
- Slice cherry tomatoes in half
- Add the above ingredients into bowl
- Add basil and garlic
- Add balsamic vinegar, and toss

HEALTH BENEFITS:
(ROMAINE/SPRING MIX)

- High in vitamins A & C which fights inflammation and boosts the immune system.

- Beta carotene has been shown to help prevent eye problems.

- Assists with good digestion, which is necessary for the production of certain neurotransmitters

HEALTH BENEFITS: TOMATOES

- CONTAINS CANCER-FIGHTING ANTIOXIDANTS

- ANTIOXDANTS ARE NECESSARY FOR A HEALTHY IMMUNE SYSTEM.

- THE LYCOPENE IN TOMATOES HAS BEEN SHOWN IN RESESARCH STUDIES TO CONTRIBUTE TO HEART HEALTH.

- A DIET HIGH IN LYCOPENE HAS BEEN SHOWN TO LOWER THE RISK OF BONE-RELATED DISEASES.

HEALTH BENEFITS OF MOZZARELLA

1. ONE OUNCE OF MOZZARELLA CONTAINS 18% OF YOUR DAILY INTAKE OF CALCIUM, WHICH BENEFITS BOTH THE BONES AND THE TEETH.

2. AS AN ADDED BONUS, THIS PARTICULAR CHEESE CONTAINS PHOSPHORUS, WHICH JUST SO HAPPENS TO BE A MINERAL THAT HELPS YOUR BODY ABSORB CALCIUM.

HEALTH BENEFITS: BASIL

1. The oil in Basil has been shown to battle skin irritations and help small wounds to heal faster.
2. Basil:
   - Contains powerful antioxidants
   - Is good for the digestive system
   - Is an anti-inflammatory herb
   - Is good for the nervous system
   - Has been shown to help with headaches
   - Has been shown to help with insomnia
   - Contains antibacterial properties

HEALTH BENEFITS: ONIONS

1. HELPS LOWER THE RISK OF HEART DISEASE
2. LOADED WITH ANTIOXIDANTS, WHICH BOOSTS THE IMMUNE SYSTEM AND HELPS THE BODY FIGHT FREE RADICALS.
3. STUDIES HAVE REVEALED THAT ONIONS CAN HELP CONTROL BLOOD SUGAR.
4. THE POTENT ANTI-INFLAMMATORY INGREDIENTS IN ONIONS HELPS REDUCE HIGH BLOOD PRESSURE AND MAY ALSO REDUCE THE RISK OF HARMFUL BLOOD CLOTTING.
5. ONIONS ARE FULL OF ANTIBACTERIAL PROPERTIES.

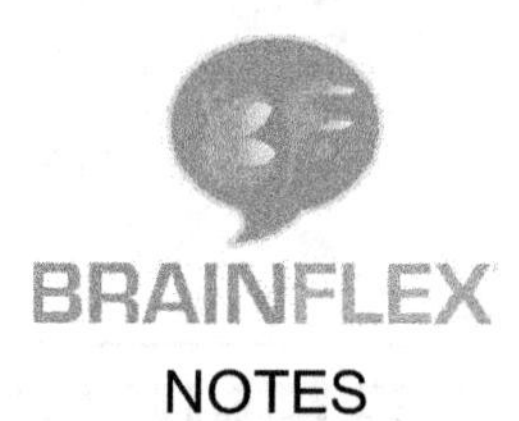

BRAINFLEX

NOTES

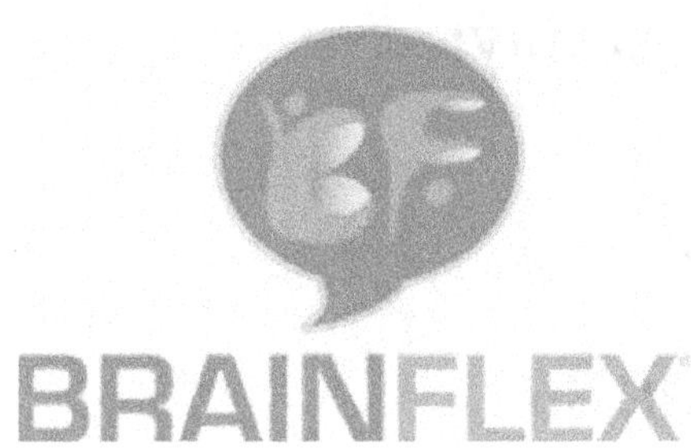

Lesson
5

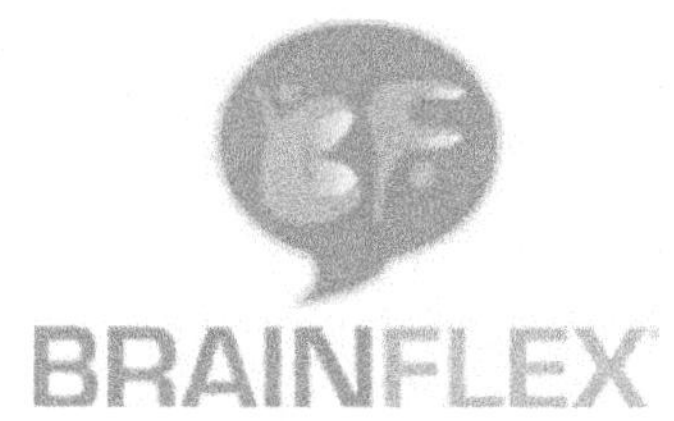

Reminder Page

Don't forget to check off the following after you complete them today:

_____ **Exercise**

_____ **Prayer/Meditation**

_____ **Self-Affirmations**

SELF-AFFIRMATIONS

I believe in personal growth, so I love to learn.

I am brave and courageous.

I am curious and creative.

God has given me a beautiful, sound mind.

I have a youthful spirit and mind.

Sharing my life experiences is one way I will contribute to the world.

Lesson 5 – Research & Discussion Sheet
Musical Benefits – Part 1
News you can use and share with others too.

1. Researchers have confirmed that our teenage brain connects us to music more during these years than any other time in our life. This complex entanglement keeps certain memories connected, and this connection doesn't grow weaker over time.

2. The 'nostalgia' we feel when we hear certain songs has a scientific 'why' behind it.

    a. Researchers call this a *'**neuronic command'***
       <u>Here's how it works:</u>
       We remember songs from our youth more than we do during any other stage of life. Why? Because, at this age, the brain is going through a very significant time of development, as is one's emotional and mental development. This is the time of life when individual's are trying to figure out who they are, apart from the parental and/or familial unit.

    b. More about the process:
       When we hear a song, it immediately stimulates the auditory cortex. Our brain quickly connects the rhythm, melody, and lyrics, cementing it to that moment. Have you ever heard the phrase, 'neurons that fire together wire together'? It's this process that researchers are referring to when they make this statement. When neurons fire at the same time, it allows them to be stored in our memory together, rather than in various parts of the brain, which is how most memories are stored.

3. Brain imaging studies have shown that listening to our favorite songs stimulates our brain's pleasure circuit, releasing dopamine, serotonin, oxytocin and other neuro chemicals, all given to us by God to bring us joy!

REFERENCES: *Article Written by*: Mark Joseph Stern is a writer for ***Slate***. Website:
http://www.slate.com/articles/health_and_science/science/2014/08/musical_nostalgia_the_psychology_and_neu
roscience_for_song_preference_and.html

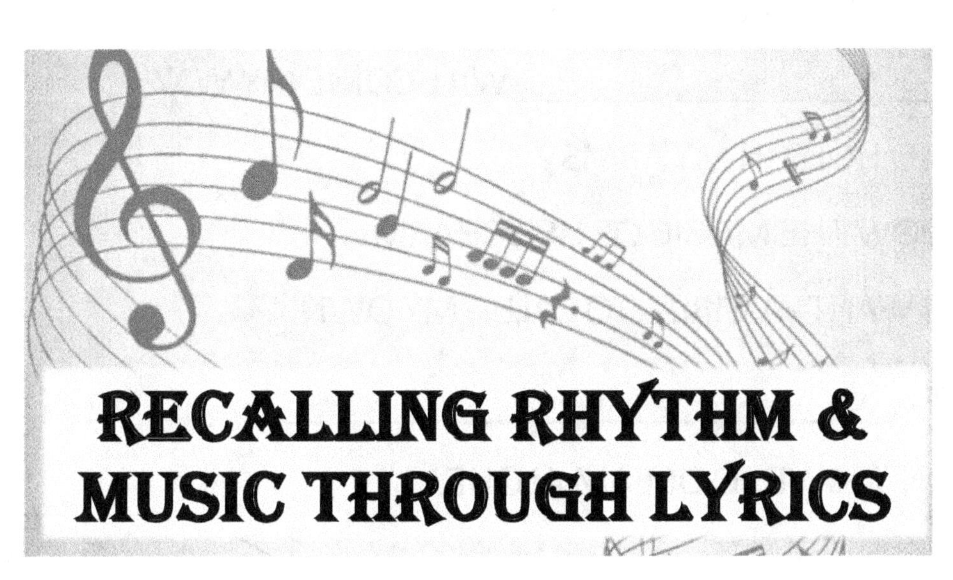

<u>On the following slides are the lyrics to the top billboard songs in 1959.</u>

-Read the lyrics and challenge yourself to recall the rhythm.
-Once you recognized the song, write the title in the space provided.
-Take some time to listen to the songs on a computer, iPad, or iPhone.

HINT: The missing lyrics are the same as the song's title.

1. ______________ ______________

EVERY NIGHT I HOPE AND PRAY

A ___________ ___________ WILL COME MY WAY

A GIRL TO HOLD IN MY ARMS

AND KNOW THE MAGIC OF HER CHARM

CAUSE I WANT--A GIRL---TO CALL—MY OWN

I WANT A ____________ ____________

SO I DON'T HAVE TO DREAM ALONE

2. ________________________

Oh-oh-over and over
I try to prove my love to you
over and over
what more can I do
over and over
my friends say I'm a fool
but oh-oh-over and over
I'll be a fool for you
…cause you've got ______________
Walk-__________________
Smile-__________________
Love-__________________

3. ___________ _______ - _______

Shoo bee doo bop, bop, bow
Shoo bee doo bop, bop, bow
Shoo bee doo bop, bop, bow

My heart is crying, crying… _____ _____ - _____
My pillows never dry of… _____ _____ - _____
Come home, come home!
Just say you will… say you will… say you will
Hey! Hey!...say you will
My heart is crying crying

__________ _______ - _______

4. _____ - ________ ____ ______ _______

When you left me all alone…
at the record hop
Told me you were going out…
for a soda pop
You were gone for quite awhile
Half an hour or more…
You came back and man oh man
This is what I saw…

_____ - ________ ____ ______ _______

5. _________ _________ _________ ______

He was a famous trumpet man from our Chicago way
He had a boogie style that no one else could play
He was the top man at his craft,
but then his number came up,
and he was gone with the draft.
He's in the army now, a blowin' reveille
He's the _________ __________ ___________
______ of ____________ ____.

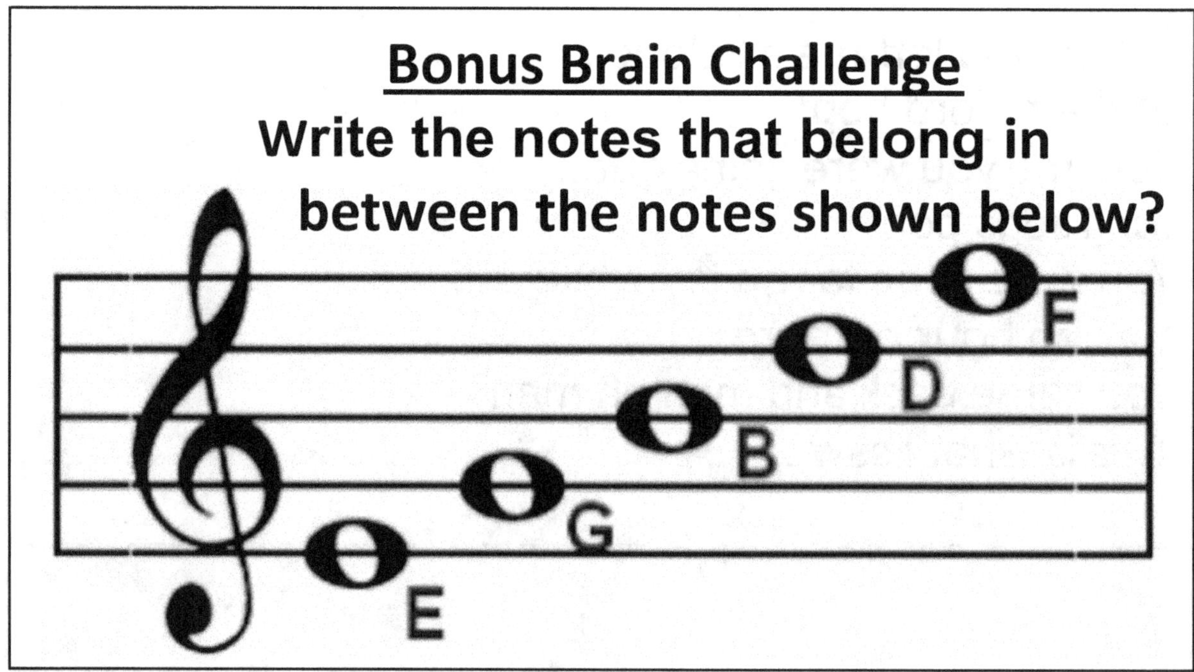

Bonus Brain Challenge
Write the notes that belong in between the notes shown below?

More Musical Knowledge Challenge

1.) In the song, "*Joy to the World*" by 'Three Dog Night', they sang of their friend _________________ who was a bullfrog.
    a. Jadzea
    b. Jeremiah
    c. Joshua

2.) The Beatles first appeared on the Ed Sullivan show on February 9th, 1964. **TRUE** or **FALSE**

3.) The all-girl group, '*The Supremes*' had 15 consecutive #1 hit singles. **TRUE** or **FALSE**

4.) In the song, '*I'm a Believer*' by 'The Monkees', they sang about love, as follows: I thought love was *only true in dragon tales.*
TRUE or **FALSE**

5.) In 1972, the 'women's movement' was in full swing, when Helen Reddy wrote a song titled, '*I am Woman*', claiming that wisdom is_________________________________?
    a. From Female Intuition
    b. Born in Pain
    c. Genetically Inherited

6.) On what floor is the apartment that's mentioned in the 'Rolling Stones song', '*Get Off My Cloud*'?
    a. 99th   b. 100th   c. Top Floor

7.) In 1964, the song '*Chapel of Love*' was made famous by which group?
    a. The Dixie Chicks
    b. The Dixie Cups
    c. The Dixie Road Warriors

8.) In the song, '*The Twelfth of Never*', to what is 'a melted heart' compared?
    a. Ice Cream in June   b. April Snow   c. Crushed Ice

9.) In the song, '*Book of Love*', the break-up occurs in 'Chapter 4'.
TRUE or **FALSE**

10.) In the song '*All I Have to Do is Dream*' by the 'Everly Brothers', they sing about 'tasting her lips when they dream'. What do they claim her lips taste like?   a. Cigars   b. Sugar   c. Beer   d. Wine

1. In the space provided below, explain how the entire triangle could be flipped upside down by only moving 3 of the 10 circles.

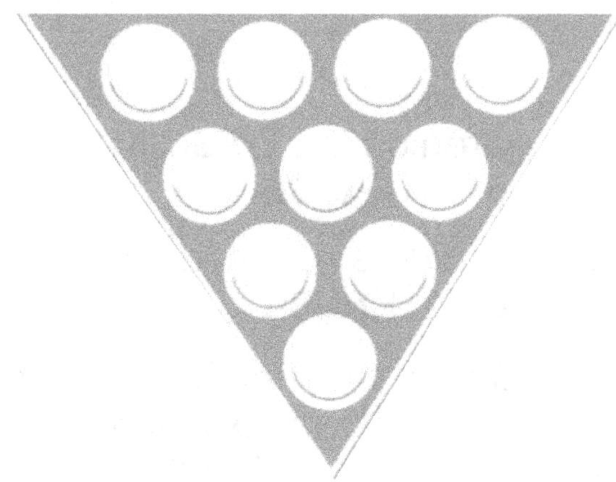

____

____

2. Imagine shape 'A' is folded into a cube. If the two dots appeared on the top, how many dots would you see on the front and on the right side? (The two visible sides) (*Fill in the dots accordingly* .)

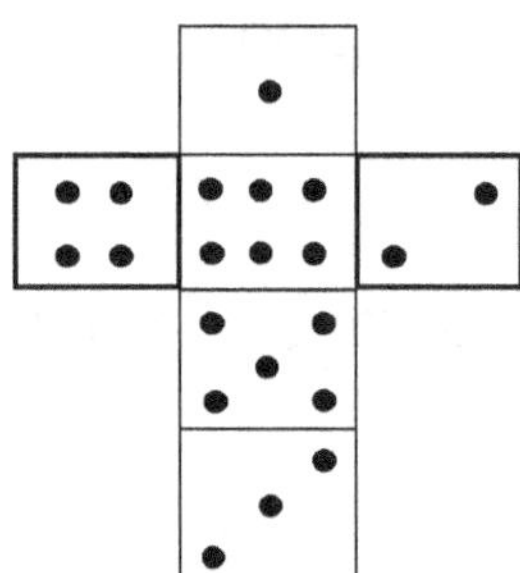
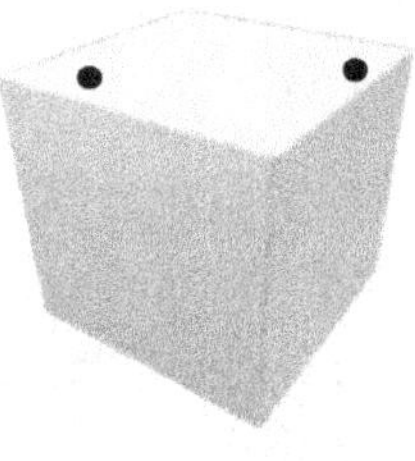

3. The following pictures only shows a portion of the actual picture. Exercise your visual skills by attempting to determine what the larger image might be if you 'zoomed' out, then write what you believe it to be in the space provided.

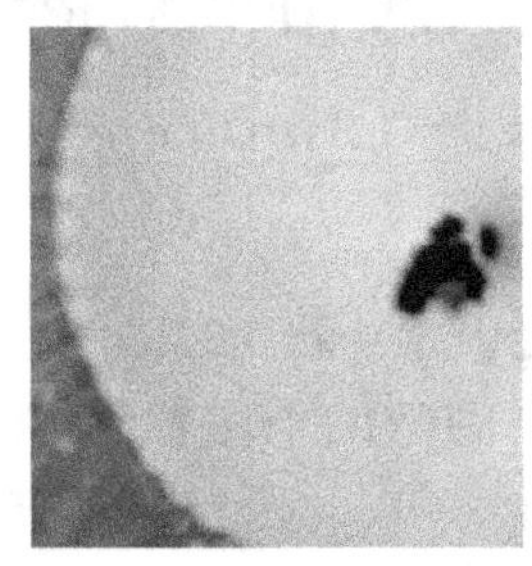
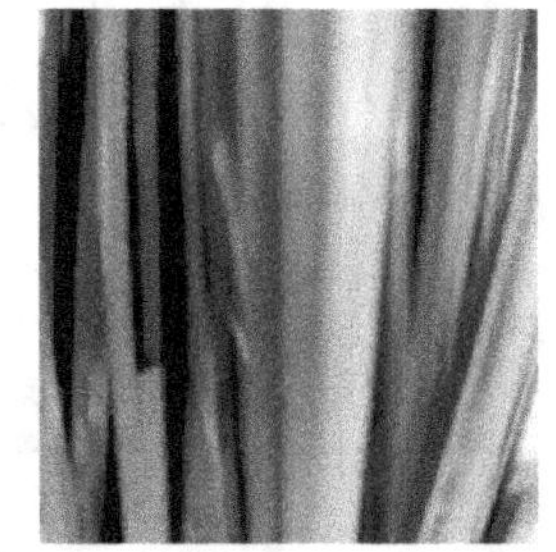
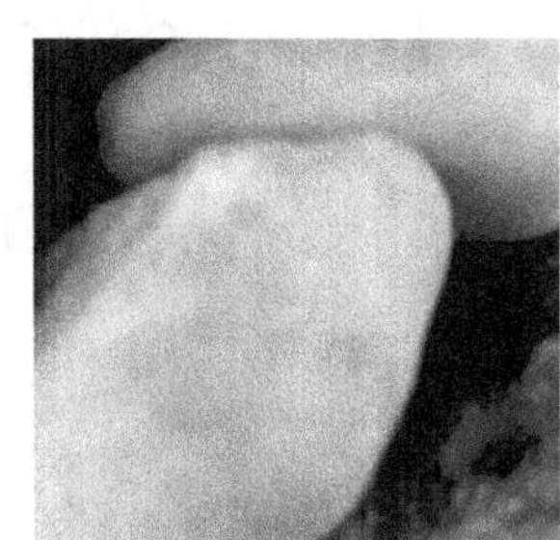

a.________________   b. ________________   c. ________________

INDECISION

In the world of indecision, I find myself at rest,
It's here I dwell most often, no longer as a guest.
Why do I seem to wander here, where all is so uncertain,
Where the mind's eye looks to nothing, or to a secret unveiled curtain.
Is it fear that keeps me in this world? Has it come back now disguised?
So many times it has been conquered, but does it keep creating lies?
What attracts me to this place of doubt, to this uneven ground I feel?
I'm searching for an answer, I'm making my appeal.
If you have come to a conclusion, if you know why I am here,
In this world of indecision, then please make the reason clear.

1.) How did this poem make you feel? _______________________

____

2.) Why do you think the author wrote this poem? What message do
you think the author is attempting to convey? _______________

____

3.) Did the poem remind you of a time in your life? _______________
If so, write about it below. _______________________________

____

Were there any parts to the poem you found confusing? ________
a. If so, which part(s)?_________________________________

____

4.) What figurative language or 'imagery' does the poem use?

____

5.) The last two lines of the poem read:
If you have come to a conclusion, if you know why I end up here,
in this world of indecision, then please make the reason clear.

After reading the poem, are you able to surmise an answer to the
author's question? Explain: _____________________________

____

Note: Sharing your thoughts about poetry with others is a wonderful
way to get to know others and can help build stronger relationships.

MATH: FOUNDATIONAL REVIEW

Math is a foundational skill, and one that plays an important role in our everyday lives. This is one reason we review basic foundational math principles often. This is a skill we definitely want to keep sharp.

$$
\begin{array}{r} 423\ 964\ 553 \\ +\ 688\ 286\ 887 \end{array}
\qquad
\begin{array}{r} 128\ 681\ 543 \\ +\ 888\ 719\ 468 \end{array}
\qquad
\begin{array}{r} 456\ 483\ 276 \\ +\ 767\ 618\ 754 \end{array}
$$

$$
\begin{array}{r} 408\ 688\ 547 \\ +\ 894\ 485\ 783 \end{array}
\qquad
\begin{array}{r} 995\ 635\ 927 \\ +\ 246\ 697\ 283 \end{array}
\qquad
\begin{array}{r} 549\ 199\ 857 \\ +\ 687\ 962\ 184 \end{array}
$$

$$
\begin{array}{r} 763\ 377\ 967 \\ +\ 848\ 932\ 294 \end{array}
\qquad
\begin{array}{r} 889\ 975\ 658 \\ +\ 541\ 379\ 948 \end{array}
\qquad
\begin{array}{r} 814\ 696\ 299 \\ +\ 195\ 468\ 996 \end{array}
$$

$15\overline{)82680}$ $\qquad$ $83\overline{)219784}$ $\qquad$ $43\overline{)213022}$

$54\overline{)107514}$ $\qquad$ $77\overline{)645568}$ $\qquad$ $40\overline{)136280}$

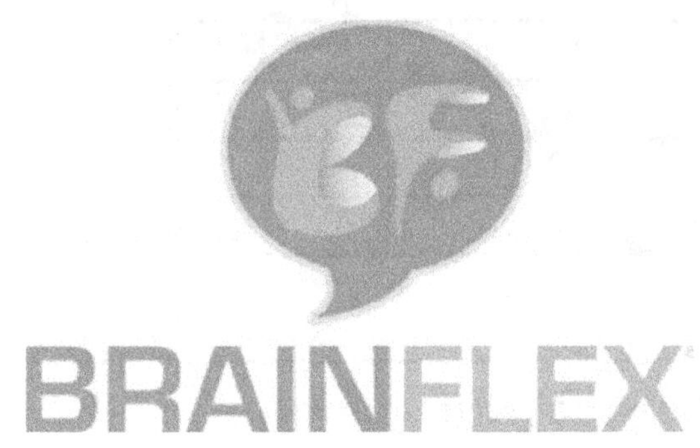

LESSON 5
ANSWERS

Answers to Lesson 5

Answers to Recalling Rhythm & Music Through Lyrics

1. Dream Lover
2. Personality
3. Lonely Tear-drops
4. Lipstick on Your Collar
5. Boogie Woogie Bugle Boy of Company B

Bonus Brain Challenge

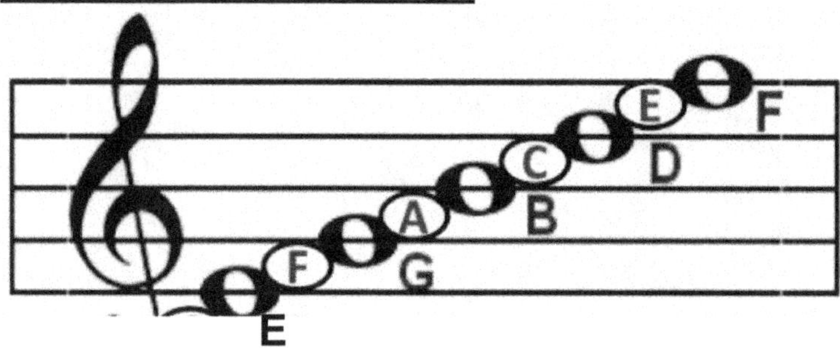

Answers to More Musical Knowledge

1. b. Jeremiah
2. TRUE
3. FALSE (5 consecutive #1 hits)
4. FALSE (Only true in fairytales)
5. b. Born in Pain
6. a. 99th
7. b. The Dixie Cups
8. b. April Snow
9. TRUE
10. d. Wine

Answers to Spatial Orientation

1. The triangle can be flipped by the following maneuver:

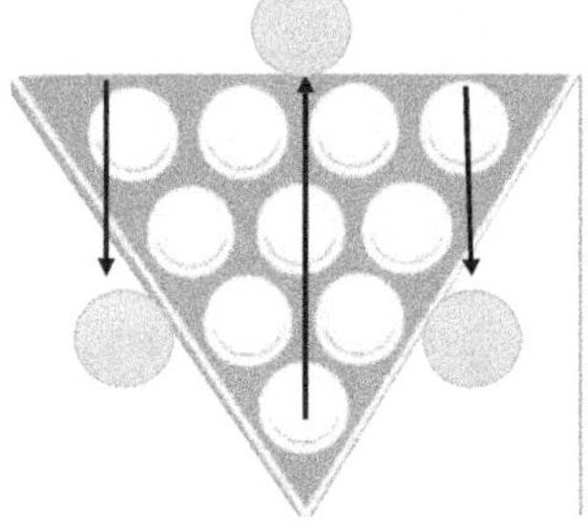

2. The folded cube would appear as pictured below.

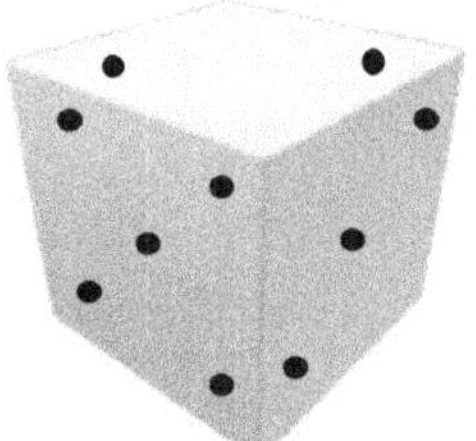

3. Items pictured 3 - candle   grass   stones

Answers Math:

1,112,251,440	1,017,401,011	1,224,102,030
1,303,174,330	1,242,333,210	1,237,162,041
1,612,310,261	1,431,355,606	1,010,165,295
5512	2648	4954
1991	8384	3407

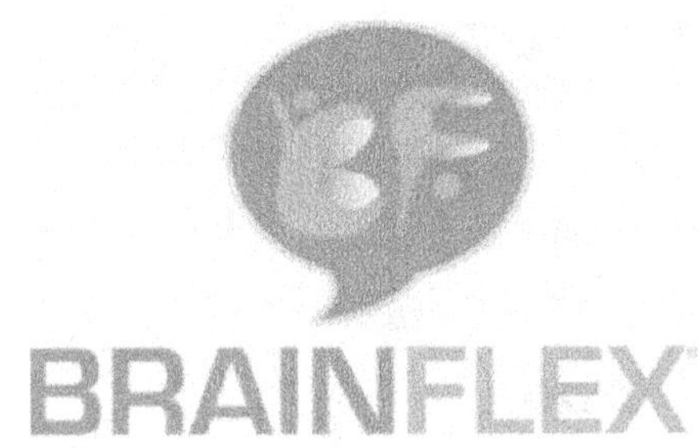

Lesson
6

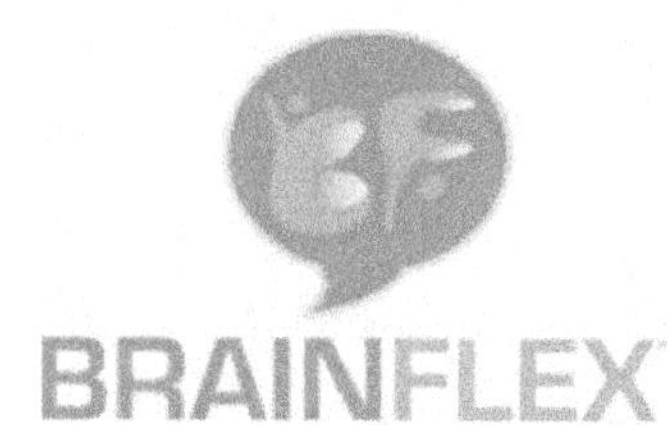

Reminder Page

Don't forget to check off the following after you complete them today:

_____ Exercise

_____ Prayer/Meditation

_____ Self-Affirmations

SELF-AFFIRMATIONS

I TAKE ACTION TO MAINTAIN MY INDEPENDENCE.

I AM FILLED WITH LOVE.

TODAY I CHOOSE TO RELEASE ALL ANGER.

MY MIND IS FREE OF NEGATIVITY.

WHEN CONSIDERING THE MOTIVES OF OTHERS, I WILL ASSUME THE BEST .

Researchers believe that the reaction we each have to music depends on a variety of factors.

Consider the following ways in which we typically listen to music, then take some time to think about the impact each of these might have had on your memory. For instance, imagine yourself as a teenager, what is one of the first songs that comes to your mind?

Now, having done that, what do you believe might be the reason this particular song comes to your mind? As we discussed in the previous lesson… neurons that fire together, wire together. During times of emotion, good or bad, we are likely to remember the music we were listening to, and as soon as we hear that particular music piece, the memory connected to it, immediately comes to mind.

Following are a few other factors that determine our reaction to music:

1. Do you sing-along, out loud? If so, you are doing your brain a big favor. How? By activating the auditory cortex.
    (This is just one of many areas of the brain music activates.)
2. Do you sing-along, in your head? Although you are firing fewer neurons than if you were singing aloud, singing to yourself still has a positive impact on the brain and memory.
3. How many times have you said, "I can't believe I know this song, I don't even like it!" This is due to the rhythm, sequence, and pattern of music. It has a way of getting in our head, even when we think we aren't listening.
4. Do you dance to music? If so, then you're allowing your neurons to get into sync with the beat of the music, which gives the brain an even better workout.
5. Do you play a musical instrument? When we are paying close attention to the words and the instrument being used, we again activate the auditory cortex along with MANY other areas of the brain.

REFERENCES: *Article Written by*: Mark Joseph Stern is a writer for *Slate*. Website: http://www.slate.com/articles/health_and_science/science/2014/08/musical_nostalgia_the_psychology_and_neuroscience_for_song_preference_and.html

<u>Christmas 'Anytime of the Year' Challenge P1: Long-Term Memory</u>

a, b, and c will provide you with the hints you need to determine the answer. Once you come to a conclusion, write your answer in the blank.

1. ___________
     a. I heard the ____?____ on Christmas morn...
     b. Dashing through the snow, on a one horse open slay, over the hills we go, laughing all the way ___?___ on bobtails ring...
     c. Silver ___?____ Silver ___?____

2. ________________(S)
     a. Many people place these in their windows, although not real, they provide a similar look.
     b. For Christmas dinner, you might place these on the table.
     c. A German tradition in the early to mid 1900's was to place these all over the Christmas tree while the family enjoyed a few Christmas desserts together.
     (They were removed immediately afterwards.)

3. ________________(S)
     a. When welcoming family into your home on Christmas, you might say, *Season's* _______?_______
     b. (Song) Mele Kaliki-maka is the thing to say on a bright Hawaiian Christmas day, that's the island ______?_______ that we send to you from a land where palm trees? sway.
     c. Christmas cards are also referred to as _____?______ cards.

4. ___________(S)
     a. (Song) Happy _____?_____ Happy ____?_____ while the merry bells keep ringing, may your every wish come come true.
     b. Some people choose to say, 'Happy ____?______' instead of 'Merry Christmas'.
     c. This well-known movie, starring Aubrey Hepburn and Gregory Peck, was titled Roman ________?__________

5. _________________
     a. The ______?_______ were hung by the chimney with care in hopes that Saint Nicholas would soon be there.
     b. You don't want to find any coal inside of me on Christmas! I am your ______?________
     c. Little items, such as candy, gum, small toys are often purchased as ________?________ stuffers.

<u>**Christmas 'Anytime of Year' Challenge P2:**</u>

Pattern & Sequence w/Long-Term Memory

Use the hint to help you unscramble each answer, then write the correctly spelled word(s) in the space provided.

1. dncay nace ____________ ____________
Hint: Looks like shepherd's tool

2. etloetmsi ________________
Hint: A Kiss

3. ahewtr ______________
Hint: Circular, hanging decoration

4. sleve _______________
Hint: 'Maker of all good things at Christmas'

5. ntsaa ____________
Hint: Chris Kringle

6. stifg ______________
Hint: '*Our finest* ____?_____*to bring* ', sang the drummer boy.

7. fstro ____________
Hint: When it's gets close to freezing, this might be seen on the windows

8. rstahsmci eter ______________ _________
Hint: Covered with memorable and/or other beautiful objects.

9. ngrmae ____________
Hint: Wrapped in swaddling clothes, lying in a ______?______

10. ho loyh gitnh _____ __________ ___________
Hint: Song: *'Fall on your knees, Oh, hear the angel's voices, Oh
night divine, Oh night when Christ was born.'*

<u>**Vocab & Language Exercise – P1**</u>

1. Begin by reviewing the hints that are given, then use your reasoning skills to determine what 7 letter word to look for in the puzzle.

(The letters that make up the hidden answer in the puzzle can go in any direction, as long as each letter in the word is in the square touching the letter before it.)

A	S	G	O
G	A	R	A
S	R	L	I
G	A	L	A

HINT: MANY THINGS I DEVOUR
HINT: I'LL EAT SOME MEAT OR I'LL EAT SOME FLOWERS
HINT: I CAN SIT ANYWHERE I WANT OR ON WHOMEVER I WISH
  HINT: I LIVE IN BOTH WESTERN AND EASTERN AFRICA
HINT: I HAVE HANDS AND FEET
HINT: I SOMETIMES SLEEP IN A NEST AT NIGHT
HINT: I LIVE ABOUT 35 YEARS

____ ____ ____ ____ ____ ____ ____

Find 7 additional words within the puzzle

____ ____ ____ ____ ____ ____ ____

2. To spell a variety of musical instruments, choose two of the partial words listed below, and connect them together.

Ban	o	pipes	pet
boe	board	Trum	Key
Trom	Bag	Cym	jo
bals	O	bone	Cell

______ ______ ______ ______

______ ______ ______ ______

In each of the challenges below, carefully study the way in which the words are located to determine the common phrase, then write the phrase on the line provided.

1) MAN
    BOARD
    ____

2)   WEAR
        LONG
        ____

3) R E A D I N G
    ____

4) DEATH ⟹ LIFE
    ____

5)   R
    R O A D
        A
        D
    ____

6)   CYCLE
        CYCLE
        CYCLE
    ____

7) [KNEE]
    [LIGHTS]
    ____

8)   MIND
        MATTER
    ____

Math Review

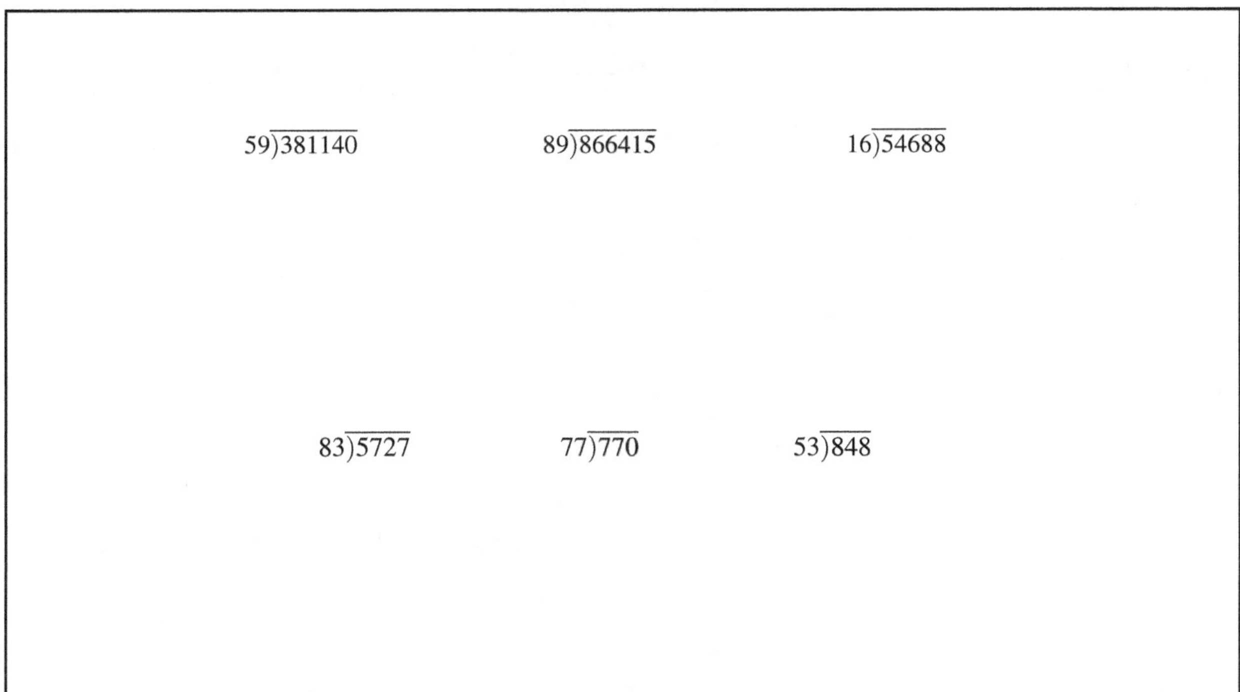

$$59)\overline{381140} \qquad 89)\overline{866415} \qquad 16)\overline{54688}$$

$$83)\overline{5727} \qquad 77)\overline{770} \qquad 53)\overline{848}$$

$$
\begin{array}{r}
937\,637 \\
\times\ 6\,185 \\
\hline
\end{array}
\qquad
\begin{array}{r}
335\,586 \\
\times\ 2\,746 \\
\hline
\end{array}
$$

$$
\begin{array}{r}
161\,184 \\
\times\ 3\,537 \\
\hline
\end{array}
\qquad
\begin{array}{r}
387\,975 \\
\times\ 6\,188 \\
\hline
\end{array}
$$

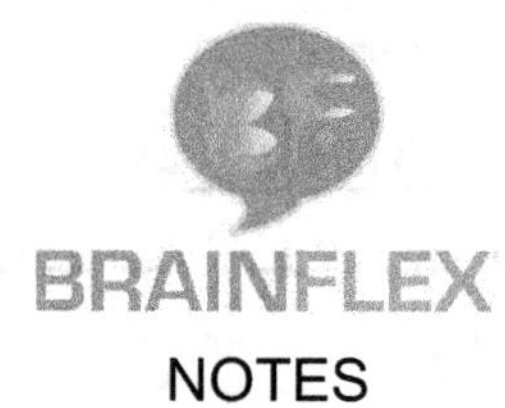

BRAINFLEX
NOTES

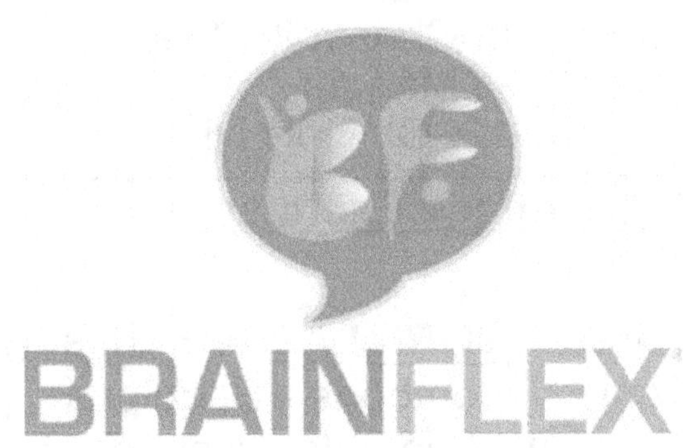

LESSON 6
ANSWERS

Answers to Lesson 6

Answers to Christmas Challenge-Long-Term Memory Exercise

1. Bells
2. Candle(s)
3. Greeting(s)
4. Holiday(s)
5. Stocking

Answers to Christmas Challenge-Pattern-Sequence-L-T Memory

1. Candy Cane	6. Gifts
2. Mistletoe	7. Frost
3. Wreath	8. Christmas Tree
4. Elves	9. Manger
5. Santa	10. Oh Holy Night

Answers to Vocab & Language Exercise –

Part 1

1. Answer to 7 letter word – **GORILLA** **rail, ill, sag, gas, gala, liar, gag**
2. Instruments are: Banjo – Trombone - Bagpipes
               Trumpet - Cymbals – Keyboard - Cello

Part 2

1. Man overboard	5. Long underwear
2. Reading between the lines	6. Life after death
3. Cross road	7. Tricycle
4. Neon lights	8. Mind over matter

Answers: Math Review

6,460	9,735	3,418
69	10	16

5,799,284,845	921,519,156
570,107,808	2,400,789,300

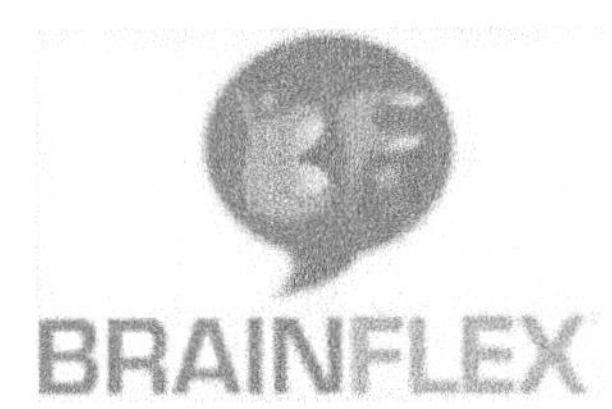

Week Four
NUTRITIONAL RECIPE

Contributing to a
healthier brain & body

The health benefits in the recipe's ingredients will vary with each individual and depend heavily upon each person's level of commitment to making healthy life-style choices on a consistent basis.

Rice Cake Supreme

Ingredients - Serving Size=1

1 rice cake

1 tbsp. of almond butter

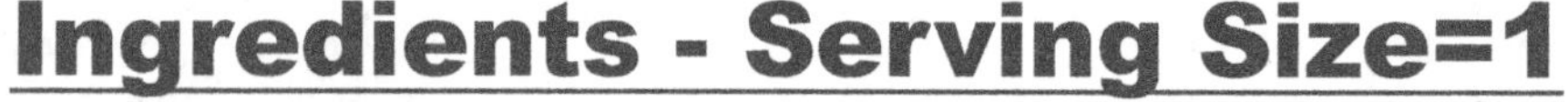

½ tsp. honey (mix w/almond butter)

¼ tsp. chia seeds

¼ - ½ of a large banana (sliced)

¼ tsp. shredded coconut

1.) Mix almond butter w/honey

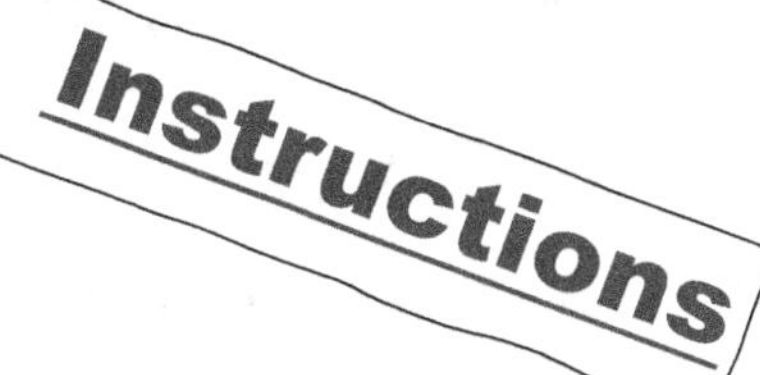

2.) Spread almond butter/honey
     mixture on rice cake

3.) Sprinkle chia seeds

4.) Place sliced bananas on rice cake

5.) Sprinkle on the coconut & enjoy!

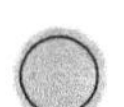

Health Benefits of Almond Butter

- High in Niacin, a nutrient that has been shown to help slow the progression of cognitive decline.
- High in protein, which helps to regulate blood sugar levels, while also keeping us full and satisfied.
- Research shows that almond butter may also help lower the risk of colon cancer.
- The healthy fats in almond butter are good for brain health.

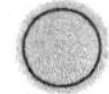

Health Benefits—Bananas

- The body uses carbohydrates as fuel, making bananas a great energy-booster.

- Potassium has been shown to help reduce muscle cramping.

- Bananas contain tryptophan, which regulates the production of seroton in, one of the main mood-boosting hormones.

Health Benefits: Chia Seeds

- High fiber content promotes healthy digestion, which we now understand, impacts brain function.
- Research has revealed that chia seeds help to reduce inflammation, which is beneficial to our joints and muscles as well as to our brain and heart.
- High in calcium, promoting bone health.

Health Benefits: Honey

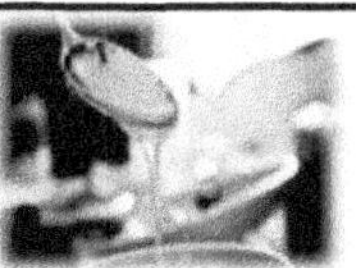

- Honey sooths a sore throat and can help reduce coughing
- Using locally produced raw honey can help reduce the effects of seasonal allergies
- Contains antibacterial properties, which are beneficial to the immune system and help promote healthy bacteria levels in the gut.

Health Benefits: Coconut

Coconut benefits the immune system, helping the body to fight infections.

Coconut improves the body's ability to absorb calcium and magnesium, which are necessary to keep our bones strong.

Coconut provides healthy fats that are necessary to brain health

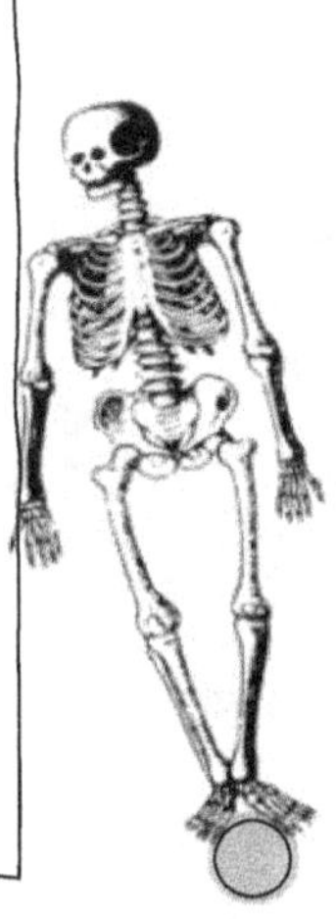

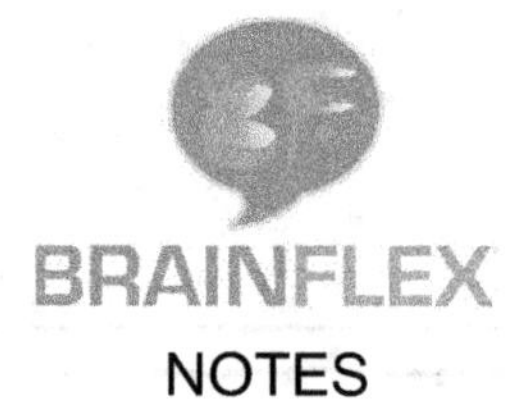

BRAINFLEX
NOTES

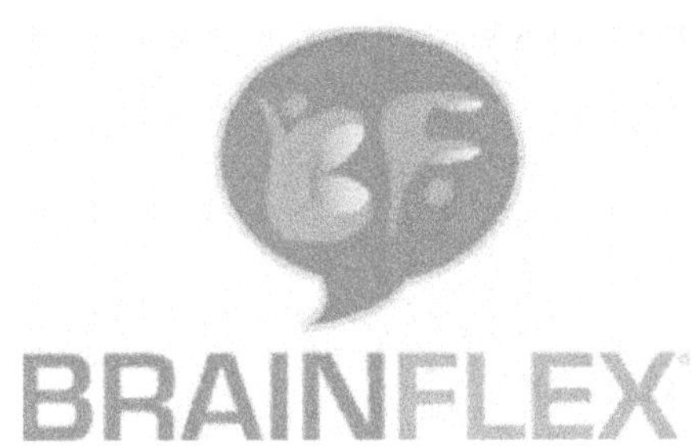

Lesson
7

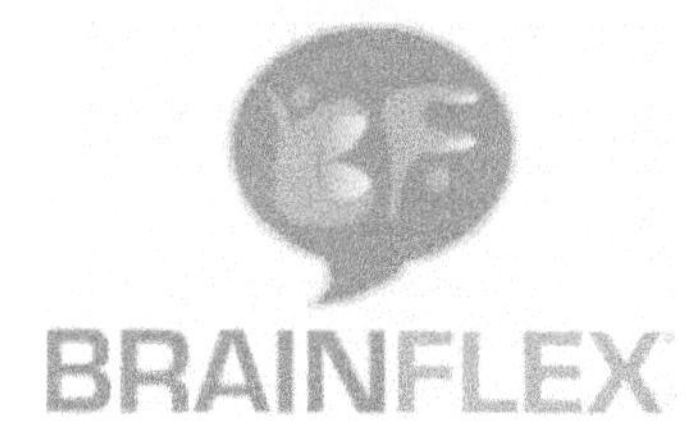

Reminder Page

Don't forget to check off the following after you complete them today:

_____ Exercise

_____ Prayer/Meditation

_____ Self-Affirmations

Self-Affirmations

I am cherished and valuable.

No one in the world has my unique DNA.

I deserve to be happy, so I choose to be happy.

I'm okay with vulnerability and I want to be real.

I talk about the lessons life has taught me with the next generation.

Today is going to be a beautiful day.

<u>**Lesson 7 – Research and Discussion Sheet**</u>
More Talk about the Dangers of Chronic Stress

Let's do a quick rundown on *chronic stress*. For the purpose of this discussion sheet, when we refer to 'chronic stress', we aren't talking about the stress that comes from one incident. Chronic stress relates to continual stress, day after day. Especially when we don't address the stress through helpful outlets, such as 'daily down time', prayer, meditation, purposeful deep breathing, stretching, and other types of stress relieving exercise.

We can reduce chronic stress by choosing to engage in activities such as these, since they have been shown to be very helpful in reducing stress and stress related symptoms.

Now, let's talk about what that stress does to our brain, mind, body, emotions, mental state, etc.

1) A few effects that chronic stress can have on the brain:
    a. Memory loss
    b. Brain fog
    c. Increased worry/anxiety
    d. Increased depression
2) How else does chronic stress affect us?
    a. Increased risk for sickness and disease
    b. Inability to sleep, which typically creates even more mental and physical issues
    c. Emotional control becomes more difficult
3) What unhealthy habits can chronic stress trigger?
    a. Tendency to eat unhealthy foods (i.e. processed foods high in sugar and carbohydrates)
    b. Temptation to drink too much alcohol
    c. Relationships can become strained due to the impact stress has on behavior
    d. We are more likely to make false assumptions or have misconceptions.
4) Additional things you can do to combat stress:
    a) Self-Affirmations
    b) Spending time with friends (positive friends)
    c) Learning new things (releases 'feel good' chemicals)

References > Alban, D. (2018, March 24). *12 Effects of Chronic Stress on Your Brain*. Retrieved from Be Brain Fit: https://bebrainfit.com/effects-chronic-stress-brain/

'Christmas Anytime'
Tune Trivia

Exercise your long term memory and fill in the
missing blanks for each of the following songs.
Have fun and release some of those
'feel-good' chemicals!

(*And it's okay to listen to the songs to help
you out with the lyrics.)

#1

Verse 1

Silent night, Holy night, all is calm

____

Verse 2

Silent night, Holy night, Shepherds quake,

____

Verse 3

Silent night, Holy night, Son of God

____

#2

Verse 1

O come all ye faithful, ______________ and
____

OR

Adeste fideles, Laeti

____

#3

Verse 1
God rest ye merry gentlemen,

____

Verse 2
God our heavenly Father

____

#4

Verse 1

Jingle bell, jingle bell, jingle bell rock

____

____

Snowin and blowin up bushels of fun

____

#5

Verse 1

Should auld acquaintance be forgot, and never

____

Should auld acquaintance be forgot,

____

#6

On the first day of Christmas my true love gave to me...

____

On the second day of Christmas my true love gave to me...

____

On the third day of Christmas my true love gave to me...

____

On the fourth day of Christmas my true love gave to me...

____

On the fifth day of Christmas my true love gave to me...

____

On the sixth day of Christmas my true love gave to me...

____

On the seventh day of Christmas my true love gave to me...

____

On the eighth day of Christmas my true love gave to me...

____

On the ninth day of Christmas my true love gave to me...

____

On the tenth day of Christmas my true love gave to me...

____

On the eleventh day of Christmas my true love gave to me...

____

On the twelfth day of Christmas my true love gave to me...

____

<u>**Logic and Reasoning**</u>

Use your creative thinking skills to consider 'out of the
box' solutions for each of the following challenges.

Jerry was hiking with his two favorite companions, 'Benny', his pet rabbit
and Wiley, his pet coyote. His backpack was stuffed full of healthy
vegetables, although Wiley refused to eat them. As they were hiking,
Jerry and his friends came upon a swinging bridge. He fastened his
backpack tightly around his waist and prepared to cross the bridge. Jerry
encouraged his friends to be brave; however, he was really talking to him-
self. They began to cross, with Benny being the first to step onto the
splintered pieces of wood that made up the rickety bridge. Just as Jerry
placed one foot onto the bridge, he heard a loud cracking sound and
noticed the ropes that secured the bridge were whipping around and
unraveling. All he had time to do was to grab his rabbit's foot, and just in
time to save him from tumbling down with the bridge.
Jerry stood, eyes wide and speechless. He was snapped back to reality
when his rabbit, Benny jumped on his shoulder and started biting his ear.
"Well, I guess we're going to have to find another way across."
Suddenly, Jerry noticed an old donkey grazing in the field a few feet away.
He immediately thought of the time he rode a donkey down into the Grand
Canyon. "Okay guys, we're going to ride this donkey down into the valley
and up the other side." As they got closer to the donkey, they realized he
was quite small. Jerry turned to his motley crew and said, "Looks like it'll
only hold me and one of you…and since my backpack is so heavy,
I'll need to take it across by itself and then come back to get each of you."

DILEMMA: Jerry knows he cannot leave Wiley with Benny, for his coyote
will no doubt eat his rabbit. He knows he can't leave Benny with the
backpack, given his rabbit's obsession with vegetables. What strategy
should Jerry use to get him, his back-back, and his animals all to the other
side of the canyon, knowing that the donkey can only carry Jerry and one
of his animals at a time? Keep in mind, Jerry will also need to get his backpack across, but will not be able to carry any of his animals with him when
doing so. ____

____

____

____

____

Exercise: Spatial Orientation, Sequence, Language and Vocabulary

Unscramble the following 'anytime Christmas' words.

sacrhtsim eter _______________ ________ *(Add lights)*

estodcrniao _________________ *(Add to the tree)*

figt pwrapngi _________ _______________ *(Presents)*

trifu kaec ____________ ___________ *(Christmas dessert)*

nstaa slucae ___________ ___________ *(Ho Ho Ho)*

In the space below, stimulate the right side of your brain by drawing a Christmas tree, and decorating it, using your 'non-dominant' hand.

Exercise Attention & Focus w/Vocab and Language

Use the letters inside the shape to form the words that will
correctly fit together on the crossword board,
with the bonus word placed in the column off to the 'side'.

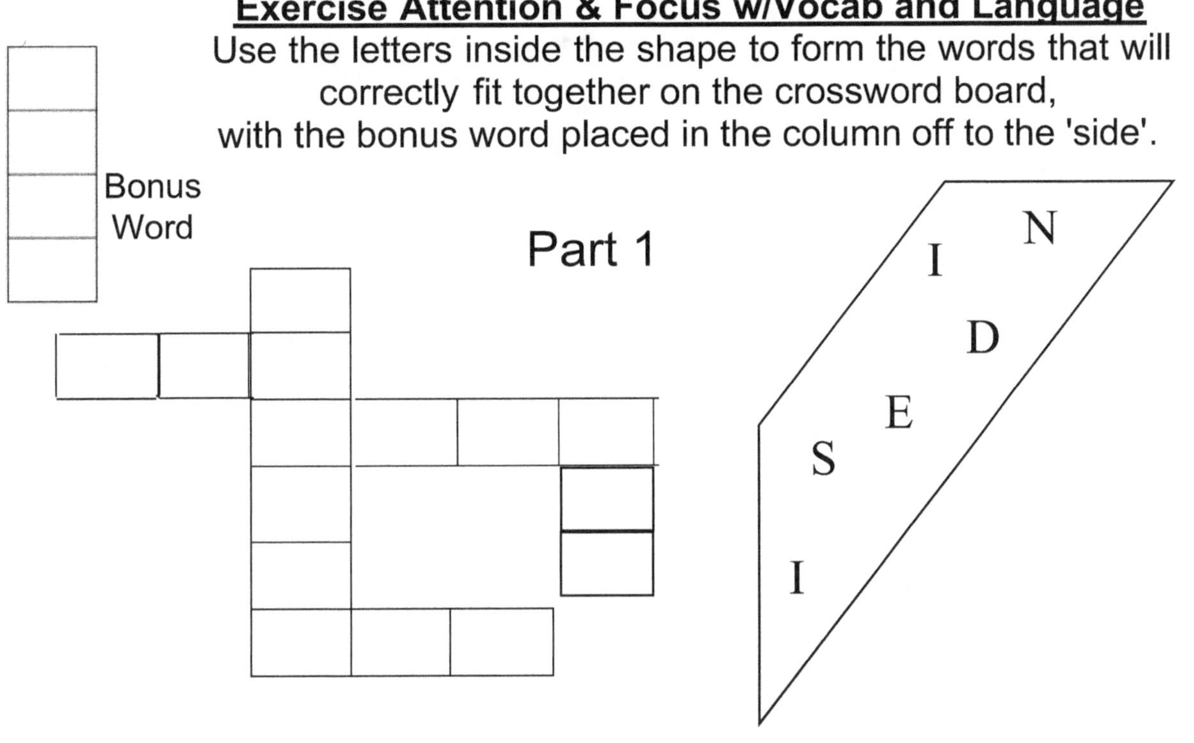

Using the letters in the shape, spell as many words as
you can, writing them on the lines provided below.

Part 2

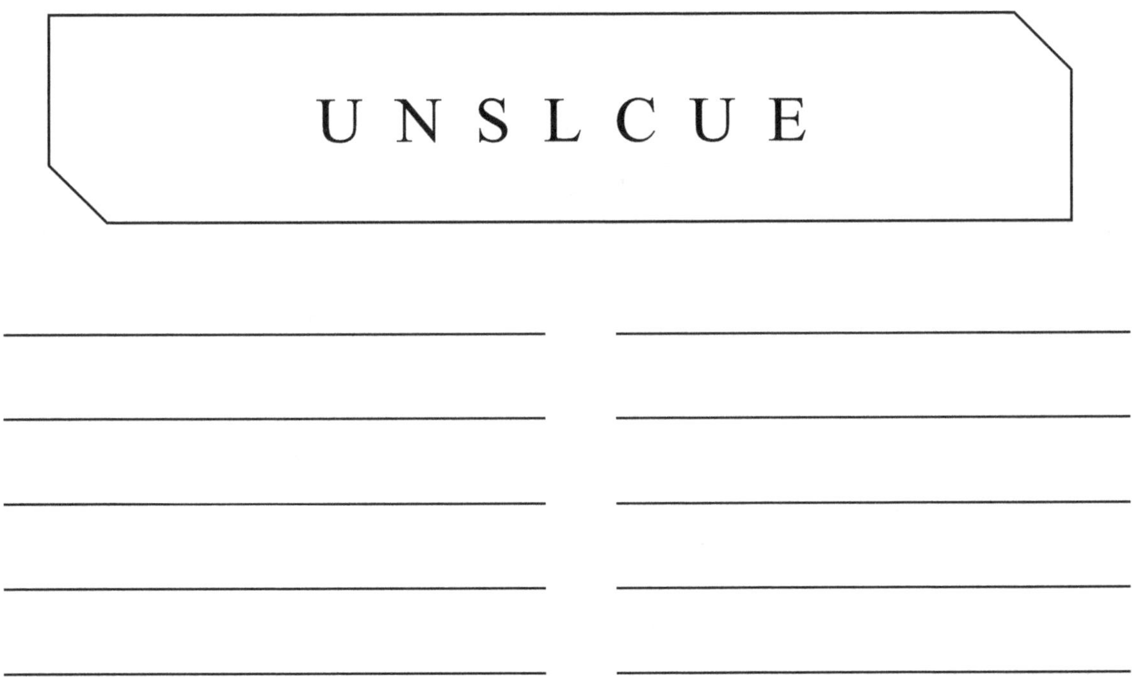

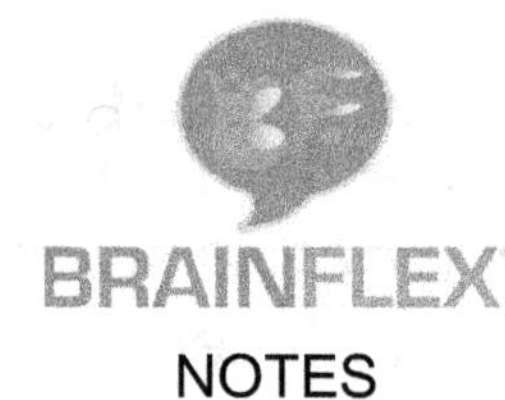

BRAINFLEX
NOTES

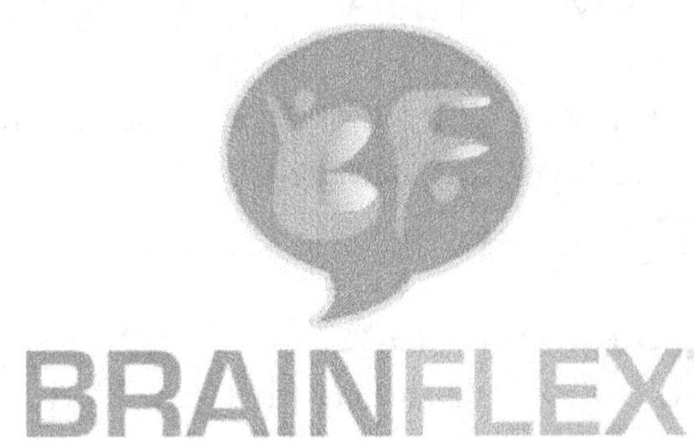

LESSON 7
ANSWERS

1. SILENT NIGHT
Verse 1: Silent night, Holy night, all is calm <u>all is bright</u>
Verse 2: Silent night, Holy night, Shepherds, quake <u>at the sight</u>
Verse 3: Silent night, Holy night, Son of God <u>loves pure light</u>

2. O COME ALL YE FAITHFUL
Verse 1: O come all ye faithful, joyful and triumphant
OR Adeste fideles, Laeti triumphantes

3. GOD REST YE MERRY GENTLEMEN
Verse 1: God rest ye merry gentlemen <u>let nothing you dismay</u>
Verse 2: God our heavenly Father, <u>was born on Christmas day.</u>

4. JINGLE BELL ROCK
Verse 1: Jingle bell, jingle bell, jingle bell rock, <u>jingle bells swing and jingle bells ring</u> - Snowin and blowin up bushels of fun, <u>now the jingle rock has begun</u>

5. AULD LANG SYNE
Verse 1: Should auld acquaintance be forgot, <u>and never brought to mind.</u> Should auld acquaintance be forgot, <u>in auld lang syne.</u>

6. THE TWELVE DAYS OF CHRISTMAS
First Day - A partridge in a pear tree
Second Day – Two turtle doves
Third Day – Three French hens
Fourth Day – Four calling birds
Fifth Day – Five golden rings
Sixth Day – Six geese a-laying
Seventh Day – Seven swans a-swimming
Eighth Day – Eight maids -milking
Ninth Day – Nine ladies dancing
Tenth Day – Ten Lords a-leaping
Eleventh Day – Eleven pipers piping
Twelfth Day – Twelve drummers drumming

Answers to Logic & Reasoning Exercise

Jerry should take Benny, his rabbit, across first then come back and get his pet coyote, Wiley. Once he crosses with Wiley, he can leave him, then take Benny back with him to the other side of the canyon, where they originally started. Jerry can then leave the rabbit there, grab his backpack full of vegetables, and take it to the other side, leaving it with Wiley, since he won't eat vegetables, then go back to pick up Benny.

Answers to Spatial Orientation, Sequence, Language, Vocab.

Christmas tree
Decorations
Gift Wrapping
Fruit Cake
Santa Clause

Answers to: Exercise Attention & Focus w/Vocab and Language

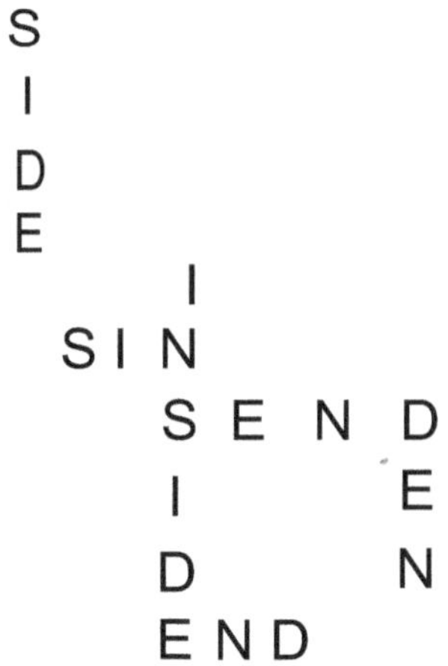

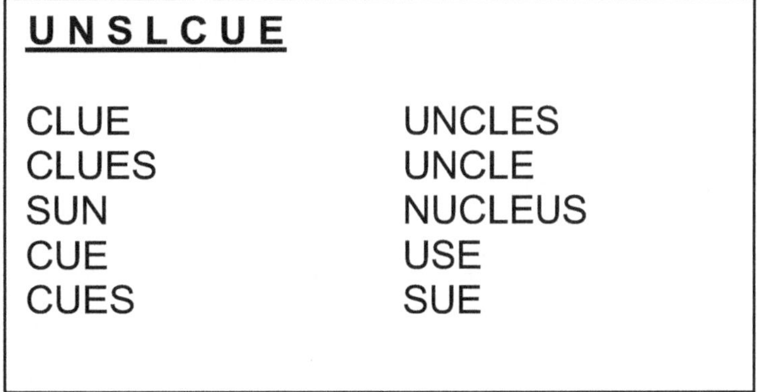

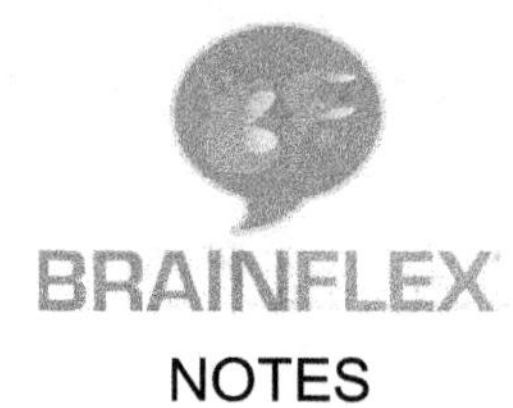

BRAINFLEX
NOTES

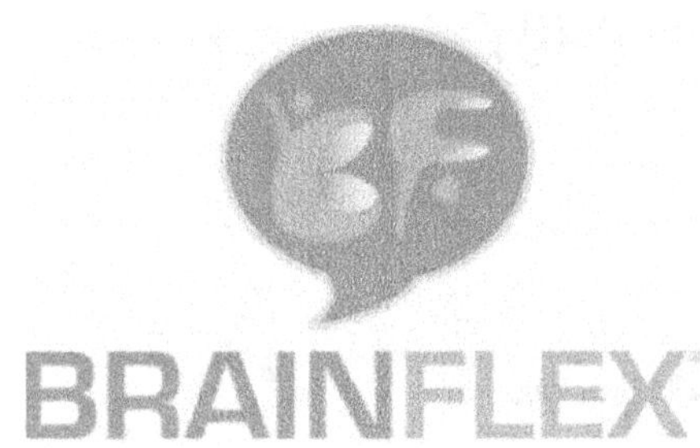

Lesson
8

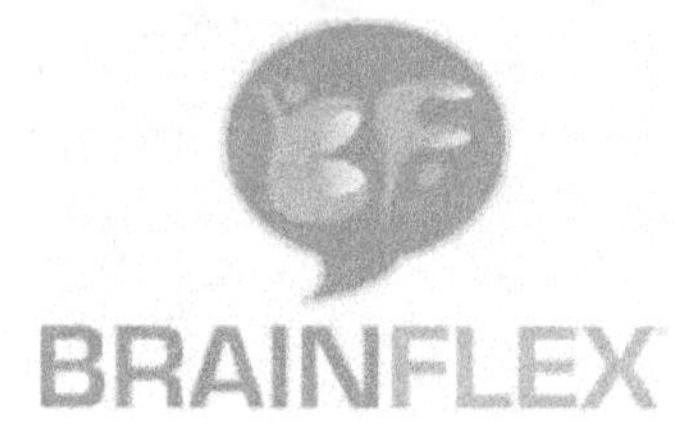

<u>Reminder Page</u>

Don't forget to check off the following after you complete them today:

____ Exercise

____ Prayer/Meditation

____ Self-Affirmations

<u>SELF-AFFIRMATIONS</u>

I WILL BE FULL OF JOY TODAY.

HAPPINESS WILL BE ONE OF MY HIGHEST PRIORITIES.

I AM BRAVE AND FEAR WILL NOT HOLD ME BACK.

I WILL ACCEPT WHAT I CANNOT CHANGE.

I WILL DO MY BEST TO CHANGE THE THINGS I DON'T LIKE.

<u>Lesson 8 - Research & Discussion: You're Worth It</u>

What if you owned a priceless, classic antique car. How would you care for it? Would you make sure it stayed clean...both inside and out? Would you drive it with great caution and only put the finest fuel in it?

My guess is that you probably answered yes to those questions...but why? Is it because it's so valuable or because it's very difficult to find others like it? Is it because it's very important to you? Or, all of the above?

Considering these things, (that add value to something like a car), how much more valuable are you? Think about it... No one else in the world has your DNA coding, which contains millions of digits and data. No one shares your fingerprint, your personality, your looks, etc. You are even more valuable than a priceless, classic antique car....because you are, and have always been, one of a kind ***and*** priceless. So, this is <u>yet another</u> argument for taking the very best care of yourself. <u>You are irreplaceable.</u>

Now that we have established that your are priceless, and you have extreme value and worth, can we agree that it's very important for you to make choices that will bring about the best outcomes?

Eating healthy foods, exercising, spending time in prayer and meditation, getting a good night's sleep, staying committed to life-long learning and maintaining good relationships are all vital to your 'self-care'.

They say that 'TIME' is one thing you can't buy… HOWEVER, if you consistently make choices that are good for your brain & body, you will be doing your part to extend your life, which is the best way to buy more time, and the very best gift you can give to those you love.

If 'aging well' was easy, then everyone would be doing it.

You can do this!

<u>EXERCISE: TIME ORIENTATION (Foundational Skills Review)</u>

Under each clock, write the time shown, (on the first line), then, on the second line, write the time each clock would 5 hours and 45 minutes later.

1. 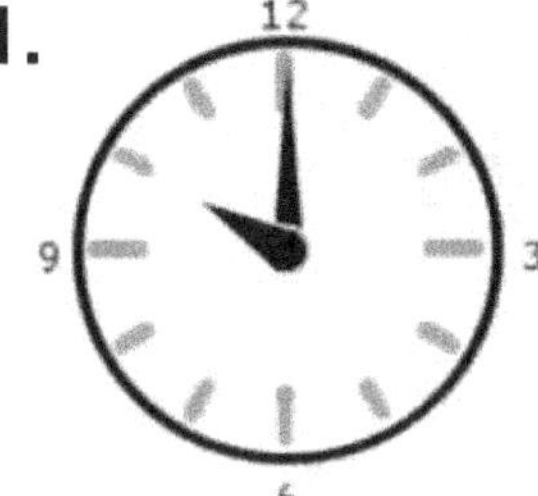

_______ _______

2. 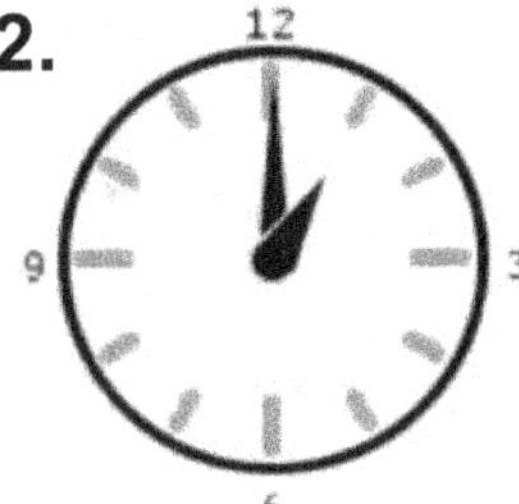

_______ _______

3. 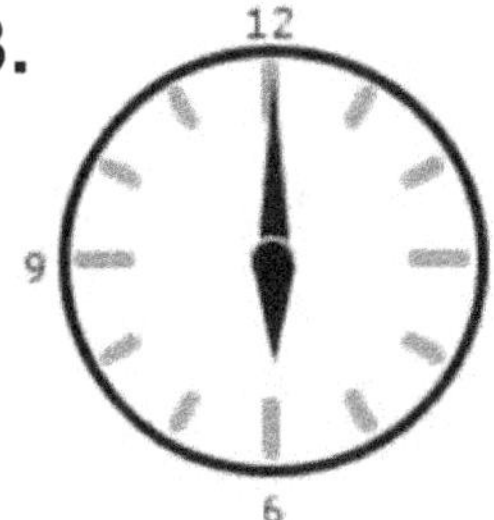

_______ _______

4. 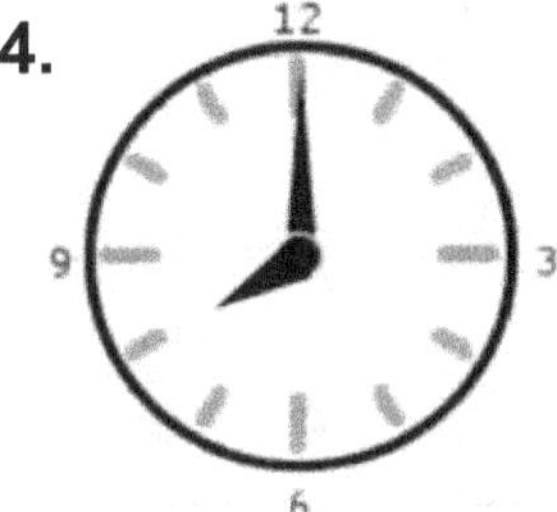

_______ _______

5. 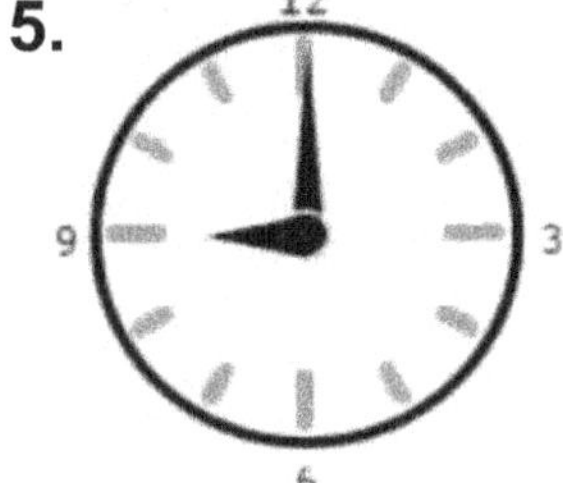

_______ _______

6. 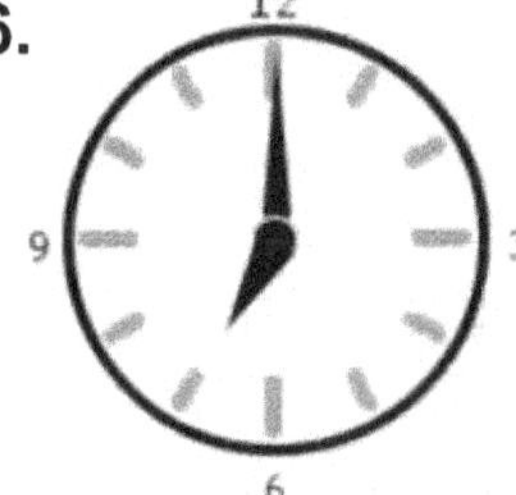

_______ _______

7. 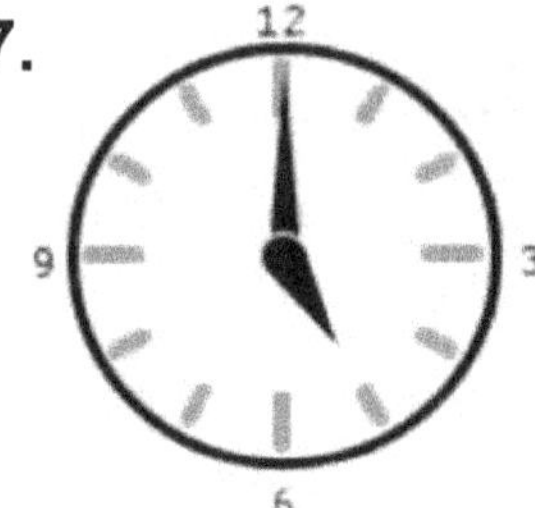

_______ _______

8. 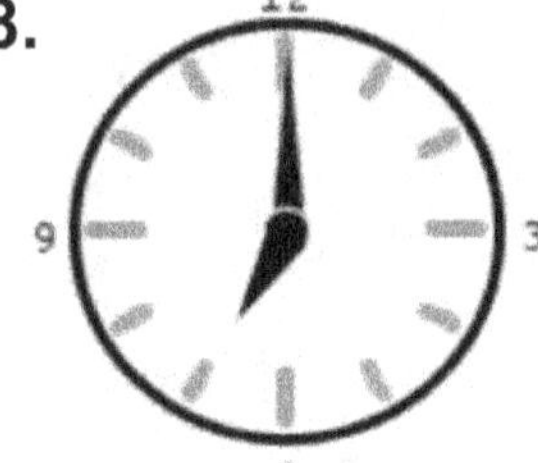

_______ _______

9. 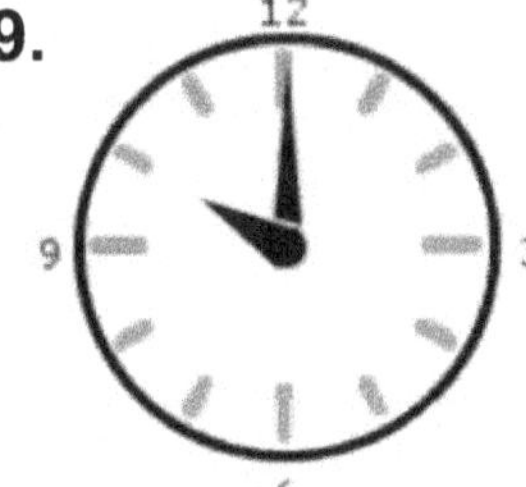

_______ _______

MATH: Foundational Skills Review

Take a quick break from the word problems and practice multiplying with decimals.

68.2 × 8.4	630 × 1.2	16.0 × 36
7.91 × 0.19	26.3 × 7.8	3.07 × 19

906 × 64	310 × 1.8	520 × 0.92
0.913 × 56	12.8 × 3.8	52.2 × 2.3

Problem Solving w/Math-Part 2

Carl receives a profit of $100 a month from one of his rental properties. He would like to open a savings account just for his rental income. There are several banks with excellent offers to anyone opening a new savings account. Review each of the bank's specials below, then determine how much Carl would receive from each bank over a 6 month time period.

Venue Bank of Tremble City -

$10 for the first $200 deposit and $5 for each additional $100 deposit

Bank of St. Charles -

$30.00 for the first $200.00 deposit and $5 for each additional $100 deposit

Arlington Bank -

$20.00 to open an account, $20 for the first $200 he deposits and $5 for each additional $100

Venue Bank of Tremble City $ _______________________________

Bank of St. Charles $ _______________________________

Arlington Bank $ _______________________________

Which Bank is offering the best deal? _______________________________

1. Find six words associated with 'COOKING/BAKING'.

S	N	E	V	O
T	O	P	N	R
P	O	A	V	U
A	P	L	I	O
L	S	N	O	P

____

____

____

____

____

____

2. Kyle is getting married today and is busy running last minute errands for the wedding. He went to the flower shop to pick up the flowers his fiance' had ordered for the bridesmaids. The total came to $176.00, which she had paid when she placed the order. However, when he counted them, he noticed they had only given him six bouquets, and he had paid for eight.

a. How much had Kyle paid for 'EACH' bouquet of flowers? $________

The florist told Kyle they would not be able to make the bouquets he was missing, and could not issue a refund for several weeks. However, to make up for this, they provided him with a voucher for 20% of any future order over $200.

b. How much did the florist shop owe Kyle for the bouquets he had not received? $____________

Later that year, Kyle ordered a dozen roses for his wife, his mother, and his grandmother. The total came to $212.00.

c. How much did Kyle pay for the flowers after applying the 20% discount? $____________

WRITING EXERCISE

Writing in cursive is extremely good for the brain.
Use this space to practice by writing the lyrics to one
of your favorite songs.

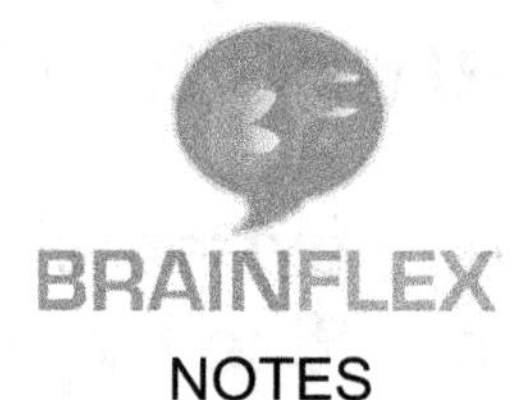

BRAINFLEX

NOTES

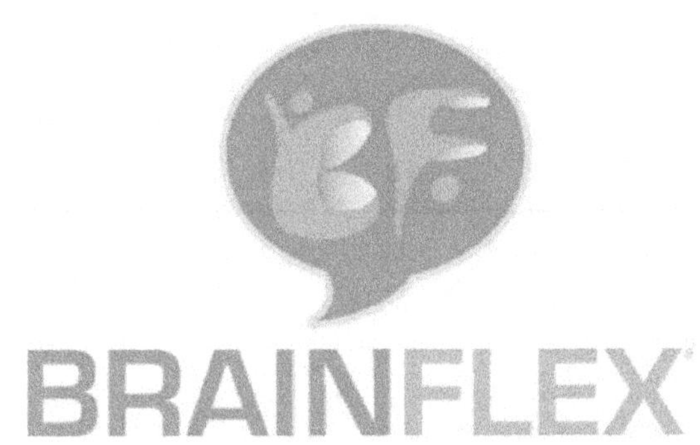

LESSON 8
ANSWERS

<u>**Answers to Time Orientation**</u>

1) 3:45 2) 6:45 3) 11:45

4) 1:45 5) 2:45 6) 12:45

7) 10:45 8) 12:45 9) 3:45

Answers to Math Review-Multiply w/Decimals

572.88	756	576
1.5029	205.14	58.33
57,984	558	478.4
51.128	48.64	120.06

<u>Answers Problem Solving – Investing</u>

Venue Bank of Tremble City: **$630.00**
If Carl deposits $100/month, by the second month, he will have
 $210 in his savings account. ($200 x 2 months = $200 + $10)

If Carl earns $5 a month for the remaining 4 of the 6 months, he will
save an additional $420 ($100 + $5 = $105 x 4 months=**$420**
($210 + $420=$630)

Bank of St. Charles $ 650.00
If Carl deposits $100/month, in two months, he will have deposited the
$200 required to earn the $30 promised for the first $200 saved,
giving him a total of **$230**. If Carl earns $5 a month for the
remaining 4 of the 6 months, ($5 + $100=$105.00)
He will save an additional $420. ($105 x 4 months=**$420**)
($420 + $230=$650)

Arlington Bank $660.00
Arlington Bank will be giving Carl **$20** just to open an account.
  In addition, he will receive another **$20 for the first $200** he deposits.
  This means that by month two, Carl will have earned another $20
  ($20 + $200 deposit = $220, totaling $240)
  $20 + $20 + $200 = $240

  If Carl receives $5 for each $100 he deposits over the 4 months
  remaining in the 6 month period, he will save another **$420.**
  ($100 + $5 = $105 x 4 = $420)

$240 + $420 = $660
<u>Arlington Bank is offering the best deal</u>

ANSWERS TO:

Exercise: Brain Calisthenics-Working Several Areas of the Brain

1. Find six words associated with 'COOKING/BAKING'.

S	N	E	V	O
T	O	P	N	R
P	O	A	V	U
A	P	L	I	O
L	S	N	O	P

P O T

O V E N

P A N

O I L

P O U R

S P O O N

---

2. The total came to $176.00, which is what they paid when they ordered the flowers. However, when he counted them, he realized that they had only given him six bouquets, and he had paid for eight.

a. How much did Kyle pay for 'EACH' bouquet of flowers? **$22.00** (Divide $176 by 8 bouquets=$22.00)

b. How much did Kyle overpay? **$44.00**

     1. $22.00 x 6 (bouquets received) = $132.00

     2. $176.00 - $132.00 = $44.00

c. Later that year, Kyle placed an order for a dozen roses for the all the women in his life. The order totaled $212. How much did Kyle pay for the roses after applying the 20% discount the florist had provided?

10% of $212 is $21.20, therefore 20% would be $42.40.

$212.00 - $42.40 = **$169.60**

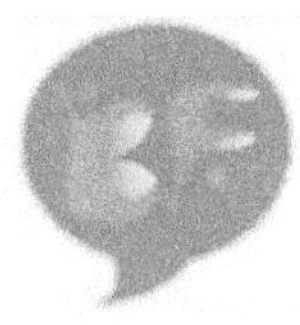

Congratulations!

You have completed the next level of 'The Aging Well' Program

The BrainFlex System
The Whole Person Approach to Brain Health

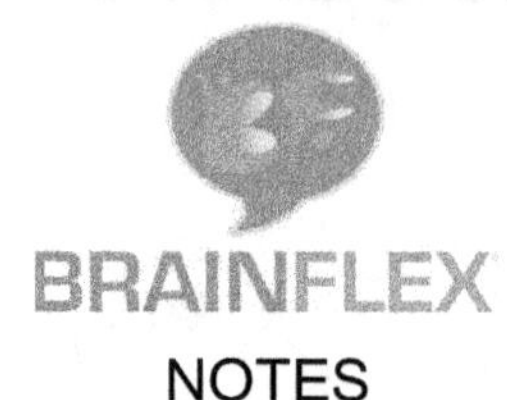

NOTES

Personal Action Plan & Wellness Notes Guide

The 'Personal Action Plan' is designed for monthly use should be used along side your BrainFlex workbook.

The 'Personal Action Plan' allows you to set goals for each of the four major concepts included in the BrainFlex system, (key components to aging well).

The 'Weekly Wellness Notes' provide a way for you to track your progress towards those goals.

This is not only a great way to hold yourself accountable, it's also a wonderful resource for families and doctors, as it allows them to read about your day to day activities and see, first hand, your strong commitment to aging well.

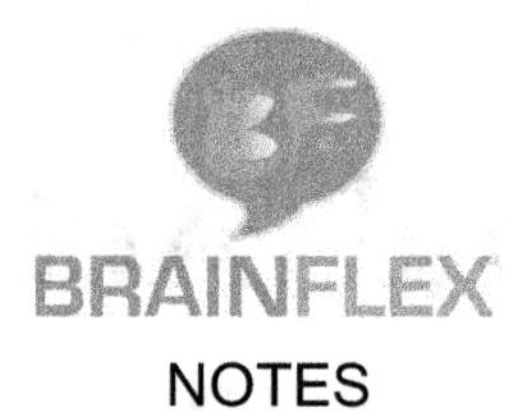

BRAINFLEX
NOTES

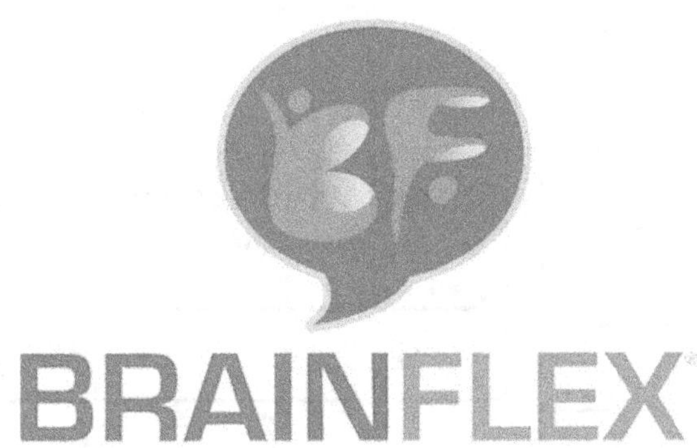

Personal
Action Plan

(one month)

<u>SOCIALIZATION</u>

Goal #1	Steps I will take to achieve goal #1
_________________	_________________________
_________________	_________________________
Goal #2	_________________________
_________________	Steps I will take to achieve goal #2
_________________	_________________________
_________________	_________________________
	_________________________

<u>NUTRITION</u>

Goal #1	Steps I will take to achieve goal #1
_________________	_________________________
_________________	_________________________
Goal #2	_________________________
_________________	Steps I will take to achieve goal #2
_________________	_________________________
_________________	_________________________

Rate your current stress level management on a scale from
1-10 (10 being the best) _________
What steps can you take to improve this number? _________________

____

____

<u>**BRAIN TRAINING**</u>

| **Goal #1** ___________ ___________ ___________

 Goal #2 ___________ ___________ ___________ | **Steps I will take to achieve goal #1** ___________ ___________ ___________

 Steps I will take to achieve goal #2 ___________ ___________ |

<u>**EXERCISE**</u>

| **Goal #1** ___________ ___________ ___________

 Goal #2 ___________ ___________ | **Steps I will take to achieve goal #1** ___________ ___________ ___________

 Steps I will take to achieve goal #2 ___________ ___________ |

Rate your current sleep patterns this month on a scale from 1-10 (10 being the best) _________
What can you do to improve in this area? _______________

____

** Watch for correlations between your sleep patterns and how often you engage in the BrainFlex concepts.*

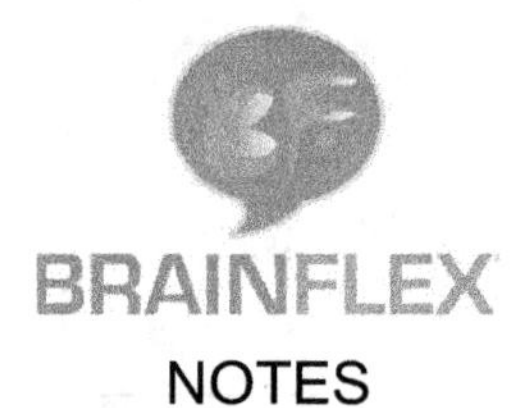

BRAINFLEX
NOTES

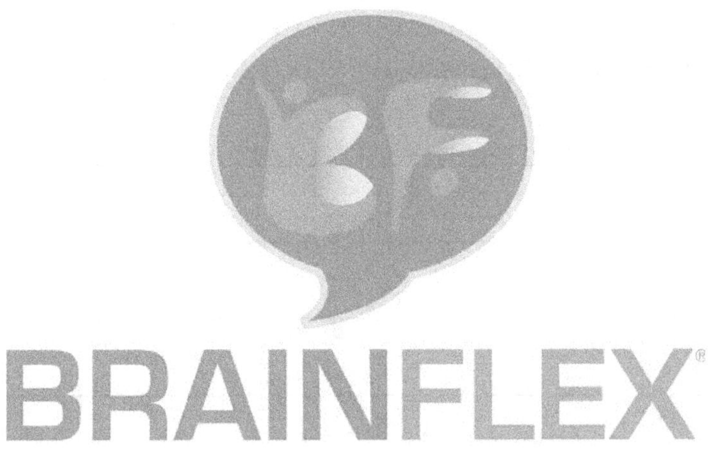

Wellness Journaling
Week 1

These journaling pages have been included in this workbook
in order for you to track the successful steps you're taking
each week towards the goals you've written in your
'Action Plan'.
At the end of each week, take a few minutes
to jot down some notes about your aging
well journey on the following pages.

Wellness Journaling: Tracking progress toward 'Action Plan' Goals

<u>Socialization:</u> How have I strengthened my social connections this week?

1.____

2.____

3.____

4.____

5.____

6.____

7.____

<u>Nutrition:</u> Healthy foods I incorporated into my diet this week:

1.____

2.____

3.____

4.____

5.____

6.____

7.____

In order to manage my stress this week, I engaged in the following...

_________________   _________________   _________________

_________________   _________________   _________________

BrainFlex® Wellness©

Wellness Journaling: Tracking progress toward 'Action Plan' Goals

<u>Brain Training:</u> Brain stimulating activities I engaged in this week:

1.____

2.____

3.____

4.____

5.____

6.____

7.____

<u>Exercise:</u> I participated in the following exercises this week:

1.____

2.____

3.____

4.____

5.____

6.____

7.____

On a scale from 1 to 10, (10 being the best), how well did I sleep this week?

Monday: ___________ Tuesday:__________ Wednesday: ___________

Thursday: ___________ Friday: ___________

Was there a correlation between how I slept and the ways in which I engaged in the above areas? _________________________________

____

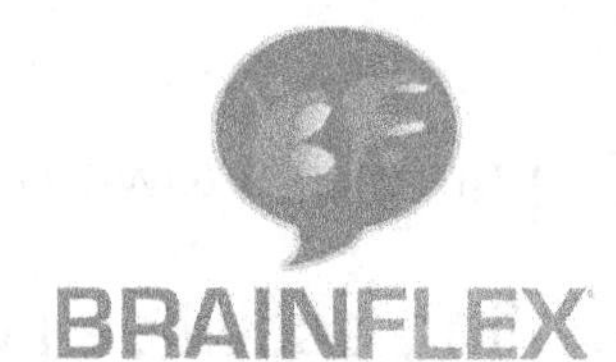

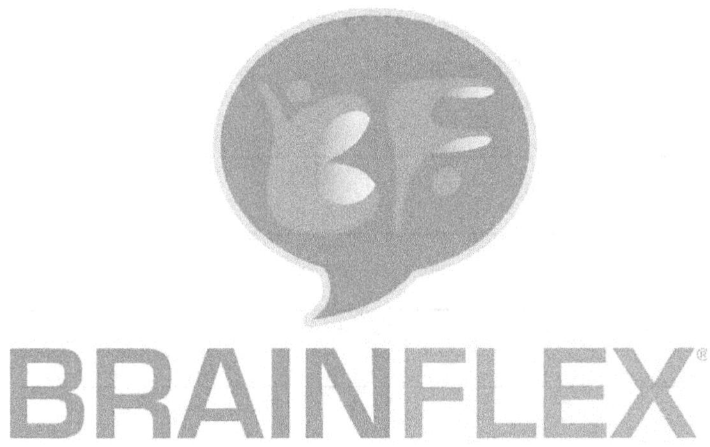

Wellness Journaling
Week 2

These journaling pages have been included in this workbook
in order for you to track the successful steps you're taking
each week towards the goals you've written in your
'Action Plan'.
At the end of each week, take a few minutes
to jot down some notes about your aging well
journey on the following pages.

Wellness Journaling: Tracking progress toward 'Action Plan' Goals

Socialization: How have I strengthened my social connections this week?

1.____

2.____

3.____

4.____

5.____

6.____

7.____

Nutrition: Healthy foods I incorporated into my diet this week:

1.____

2.____

3.____

4.____

5.____

6.____

7.____

In order to manage my stress this week, I engaged in the following...

_________________   _________________   _________________

_________________   _________________   _________________

Wellness Journaling: Tracking progress toward 'Action Plan' Goals

Brain Training: Brain stimulating activities I engaged in this week:

1.____

2.____

3.____

4.____

5.____

6.____

7.____

Exercise: I participated in the following exercises this week:

1.____

2.____

3.____

4.____

5.____

6.____

7.____

On a scale from 1 to 10, (10 being the best), how well did I sleep this week?

Monday: ______________ Tuesday:____________ Wednesday: _____________

Thursday: ______________ Friday: _____________

Was there a correlation between how I slept and the ways in which I engaged in the above areas? ________________________________

____

BrainFlex® Wellness©

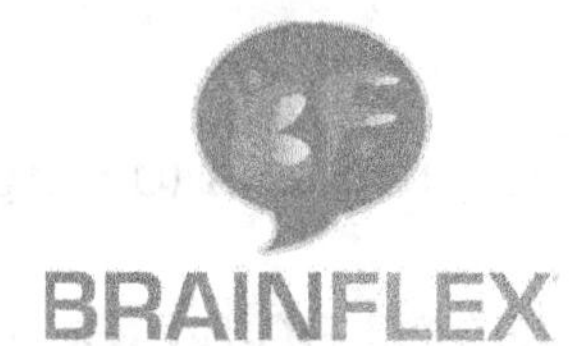

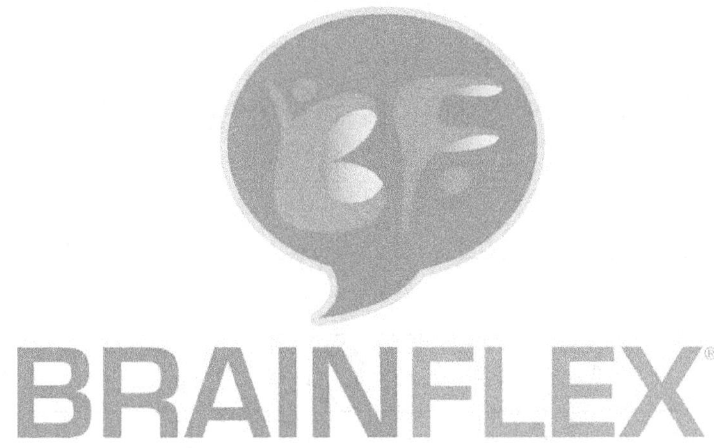

Wellness Journaling

Week 3

These journaling pages have been included in this workbook in order for you to track the successful steps you're taking each week towards the goals you've written in your **'Action Plan'**.
At the end of each week, take a few minutes to jot down some notes about your aging well journey on the following pages.

Wellness Journaling: Tracking progress toward 'Action Plan' Goals

<u>Socialization</u>: How have I strengthened my social connections this week?

1.____

2.____

3.____

4.____

5.____

6.____

7.____

<u>Nutrition</u>: Healthy foods I incorporated into my diet this week:

1.____

2.____

3.____

4.____

5.____

6.____

7.____

In order to manage my stress this week, I engaged in the following...

________________ ________________ ________________

________________ ________________ ________________

BrainFlex® Wellness©

Wellness Journaling: Tracking progress toward 'Action Plan' Goals

Brain Training: Brain stimulating activities I engaged in this week:

1.____

2.____

3.____

4.____

5.____

6.____

7.____

Exercise: I participated in the following exercises this week:

1.____

2.____

3.____

4.____

5.____

6.____

7.____

On a scale from 1 to 10, (10 being the best), how well did I sleep this week?

Monday: ______________ Tuesday:____________ Wednesday: _____________

Thursday: ______________ Friday: ____________

Was there a correlation between how I slept and the ways in which I engaged in the above areas? ________________________________

____

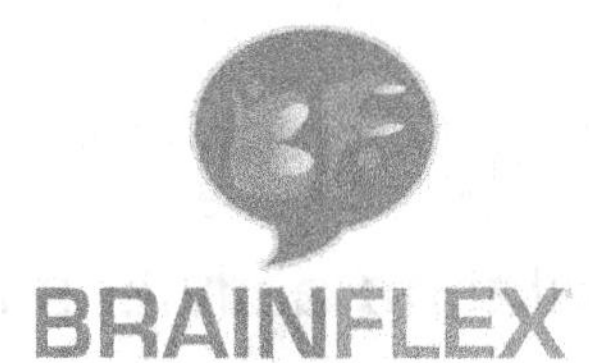

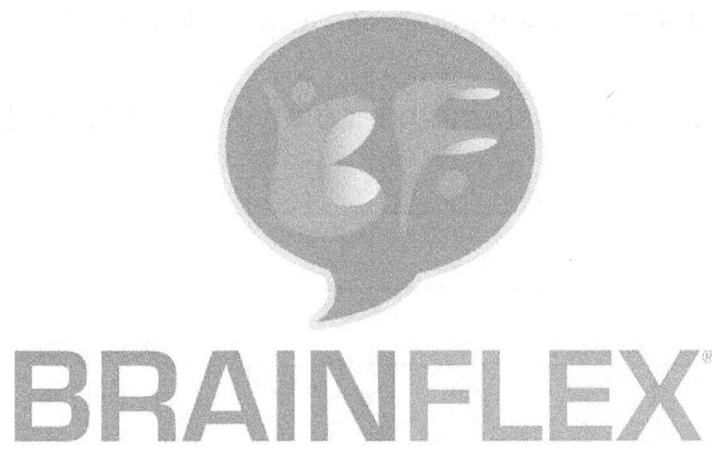

Wellness Journaling
Week 4

These journaling pages have been included in this workbook
in order for you to track the successful steps you're taking
each week towards the goals you've written in your
'Action Plan'.
At the end of each week, take a few minutes
to jot down some notes about your aging well
journey on the following pages.

Wellness Journaling: Tracking progress toward 'Action Plan' Goals

<u>Socialization</u>: How have I strengthened my social connections this week?

1.____

2.____

3.____

4.____

5.____

6.____

7.____

<u>Nutrition</u>: Healthy foods I incorporated into my diet this week:

1.____

2.____

3.____

4.____

5.____

6.____

7.____

In order to manage my stress this week, I engaged in the following...

_______________ _______________ _______________

_______________ _______________ _______________

BrainFlex® Wellness©

Wellness Journaling: Tracking progress toward 'Action Plan' Goals

Brain Training: Brain stimulating activities I engaged in this week:

1.____

2.____

3.____

4.____

5.____

6.____

7.____

Exercise: I participated in the following exercises this week:

1.____

2.____

3.____

4.____

5.____

6.____

7.____

On a scale from 1 to 10, (10 being the best), how well did I sleep this week?

Monday: ____________ Tuesday:___________ Wednesday: ____________

Thursday: ____________ Friday: ____________

Was there a correlation between how I slept and the ways in which I engaged in the above areas? _______________________________
____

BrainFlex® Wellness©

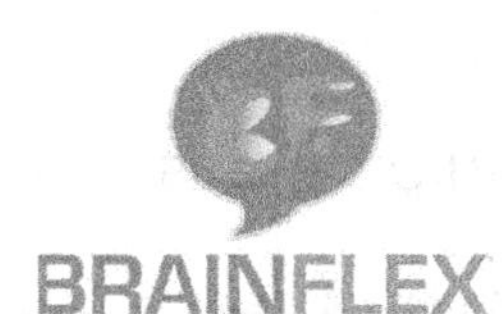

aging Well
from the experts...

Tips for Successful Aging by Rosemary Laird, MD

1.) Stay Sharp!

Keeping mentally sharp as we age is something we all want. No one wants to lose the independence that comes with a sound mind. While genetic predisposition controls some of how our brains age, there are several key areas we can control that can help our brains stay healthy and keep those senior moments at bay.

- Get 30 minutes of moderate physical activity each day
- Keep blood pressure and blood sugar in the normal ranges
- Follow the MIND and/or Mediterranean diets
- Keep cognitively active – be a lifelong learner and stay engaged in life
- Don't smoke

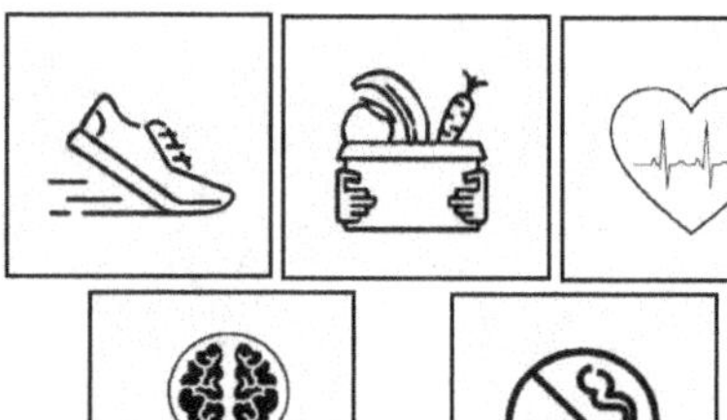

2.) Steady as You Go!

One of the earliest signs of a body slowing down and aging is when muscles become weak. When weakness affects the legs, an individual will find it harder to get up out of their chair. They will spend more of each day sitting and become less mobile. This will lead to lower endurance and decreased overall ability to walk, which then makes them weaker, and the continuous downward spiral is set. This weakness also increases the risk of falls and injury which only adds to the decline in ability.

One of the best ways to avoid this is to keep moving and plan 30 minutes of a moderately rigorous activity each day. Move it or lose it is very true!

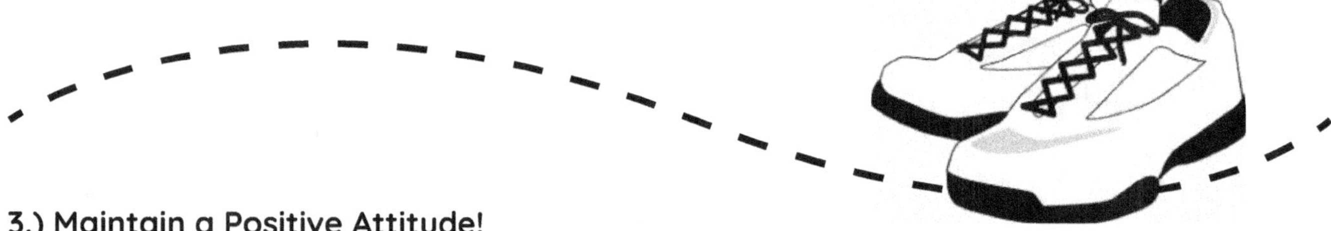

3.) Maintain a Positive Attitude!

Keeping a positive attitude as you get older may seem like a tall order, but it has a big payout. Research has shown a direct correlation between a positive attitude about aging during midlife being linked to people with delays in some of the common changes of aging such as cognitive decline, heart problems, and longevity. Other research has shown that a positive attitude is related to lower overall stress levels and that leads to a healthier state for your mind and body, so smile and remember "It's all in your head."

Scan the QR code with your phone camera to view another resource about maintaining a positive mindset.

Dr. Rosemary Laird's Tips to Successful Aging

4.) Stay Self-Assured Through It All!

Adaptation and resilience are two key attributes to aging successfully. Being able to adapt to changes in your body can mean the difference between continuing to thrive or starting down a path of decline. Here are two examples of common age-related conditions that could negatively impact your daily quality of life unless you keep a positive mindset and learn all you can about how to adapt.

- Hearing loss: Don't get left out of the conversation! Staying engaged and involved with others is a key component of healthy and successful aging. Hearing loss is one of the most common age-related challenges we all face to some degree. If it begins to impact your ability to interact with others, that's a strong indication that you need to seek help. If you answer YES to any of the following questions please schedule an appointment for a hearing evaluation:

  1) Are you having hearing problems when visiting with family and friends?
  2) Do you fear meeting new people due to a hearing problem?
  3) Does a hearing problem cause you to have arguments with family or friends?

- Urinary incontinence: Don't miss the party! This is perhaps the most embarrassing of the changes that can come as we age. We get it, we really do! The good news is there is often a lot you can do to reduce urinary incontinence and manage it discreetly. Don't let this get you down. Make an appointment to talk with your primary care provider or gynecologist. Also, check out the Seni website, www.seni-usa.com. You will find helpful information about what causes urinary incontinence, what to talk to your doctor about, and strategies and products you can use to help keep urinary incontinence from causing you to miss out on life.

Scan the QR code to learn more!

This pro-**active** approach will help you face and adapt to the common challenges of aging.

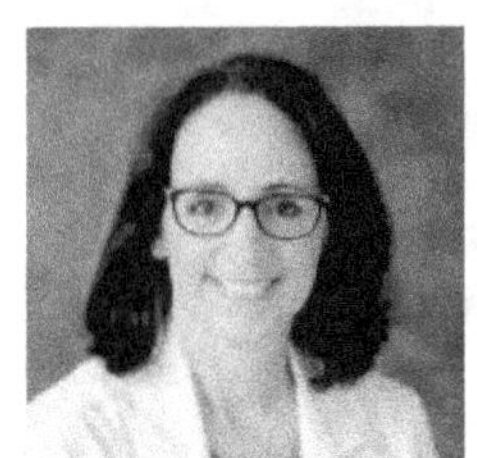

Rosemary Laird, M.D., M.H.S.A is a Clinical Associate Professor in the Department of Geriatrics at the Florida State University School of Medicine. Dr. Laird also now serves as a Principal Investigator for ClinCloudResearch in Viera, Florida. Dr. Laird received her medical degree with honors from Georgetown University School of Medicine in 1991. She completed an Internal Medicine residency and Geriatric Fellowship. She is a recognized expert in diagnosing and caring for patients with Alzheimer's disease and spent 20 years as the Medical Director for two state-designated Memory Disorder Clinics. In 2019, the governor of Florida appointed her to serve on the state's Alzheimer's Disease Advisory Committee. Dr. Laird is a sought-after speaker, educator, author and named the American Geriatrics Society's Geriatrician of the Year in 2013. She has guided the development of educational programs for lay and professional audiences, covering various topics related to Alzheimer's disease, other common conditions of aging, and family caregiving. She is a passionate advocate for the support of family caregivers and co-authored the book *Take Your Oxygen First: Preserving Your Health and Happiness While Caring for a Loved One with Alzheimer's Disease*. Dr. Laird is also a co-author with the late Fred Lee of *Beyond Disney: Heartwiring Healthcare Excellence*. She speaks to healthcare providers about this **novel approach** of infusing the heart of medical practice into the challenging world of clinical medicine.

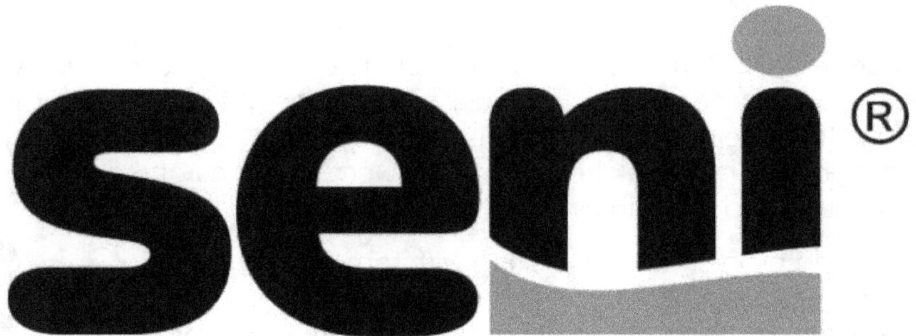

We want to thank our sponsor, Seni®, for their contribution to the *Aging Well* journey! As international experts in managing the challenges of urinary incontinence, Seni® shares our *whole person* philosophy and understands how the many physical changes of aging and common illnesses can have a tremendous impact on independence and overall quality of life. If there comes a time when incontinence holds you back, you can have confidence in turning to Seni®.

Your brain will thank you!

To Find the Right Product, Think seni®

S is for Size

Waist/Hip measurement is important. Weight will not give sufficient information to determine the right size

*if measurements are in one range, pick the size this range indicates

*If measurements are in two different ranges, defer to the larger size.

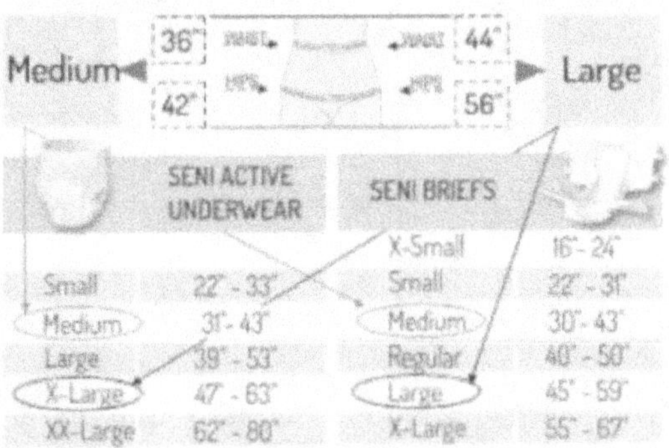

	SENI ACTIVE UNDERWEAR	SENI BRIEFS	
		X-Small	16" - 24"
Small	22" - 33"	Small	22" - 31"
Medium	31" - 43"	Medium	30" - 43"
Large	39" - 53"	Regular	40" - 50"
X-Large	47" - 63"	Large	45" - 59"
XX-Large	62" - 80"	X-Large	55" - 67"

E is for Essential Features, Evaluate Mobility, and Ensure Correct Style

Essential Features:

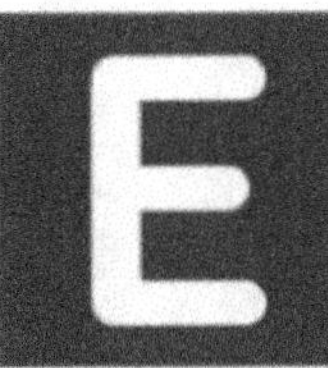 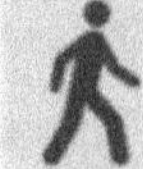 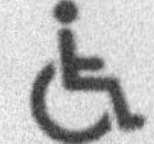 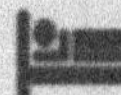 Fully Breathable Outer Layer

 Superabsorbency

Hydrophobic Standing Side Gathers

Extra Dry System - soft non-woven layer

Evaluate Mobility

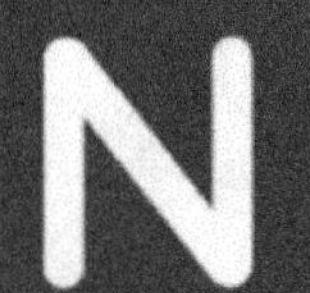
- Pads/Guards
- Underwear
- Shaped Pads

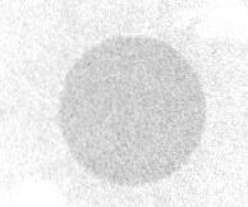
- Briefs
- Shaped Pads

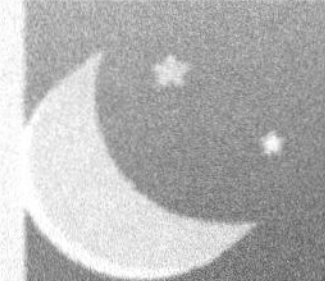
- Briefs
- Shaped Pads

Ensure Correct Style

Pads, Active Underwear, and Shaped Pads Day are ideal for someone with light to moderate incontinence. High Absorbency Underwear, Briefs, & Shaped Pads Night are ideal for someone with heavy/severe incontinence

ⓘ Underwear is a better style for dementia patients because they look and feel more like regular undergarments

ⓘ Man Fit guards are ideal for after prostate surgery

ⓘ Shaped pads are ideal for bariatric patients or those who fall in between sizes

N is for Night vs. Day Products

Sleep is valuable. Restorative sleep will help reduce the risk of falls at night and help you be more alert during the day.

For daily use, choose products that are comfortable, easy to change, and at the right absorbency level.

For overnight, choose products with high absorbency to allow for uninterrupted sleep.

I is for Improve your Continence whenever Possible

See what other factors may influence each person's individual product assessment.

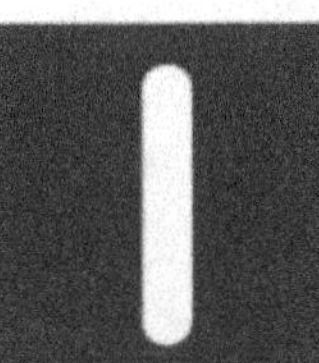
Avoid blockages to and from the bathroom. Adjust the environment for easy access.

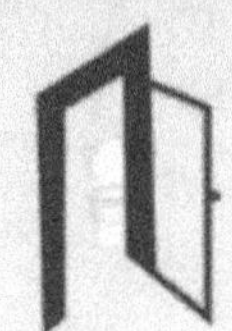
Recommend or perform Kegel exercises to strengthen pelvic floor muscles.

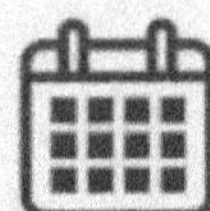
Create a personalized toileting schedule

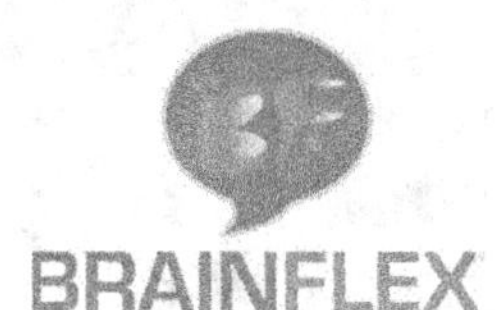

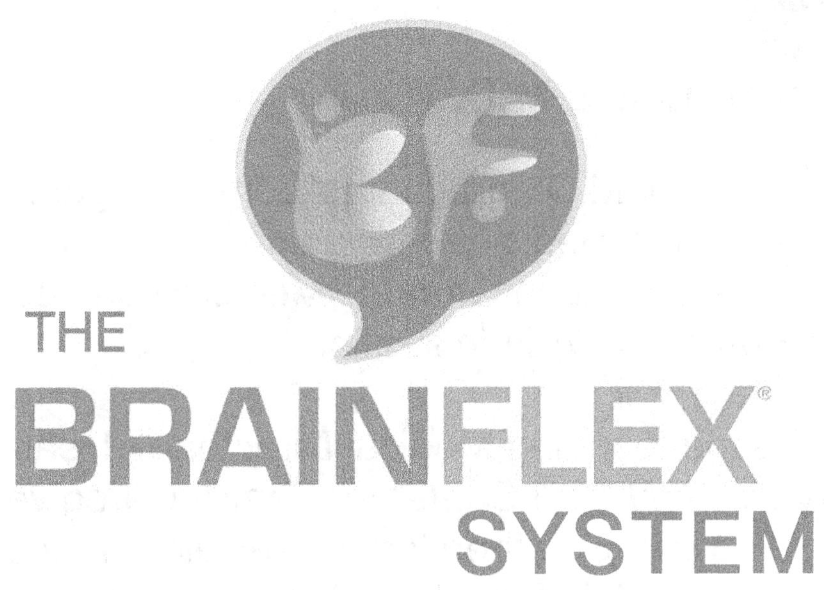

ABOUT US

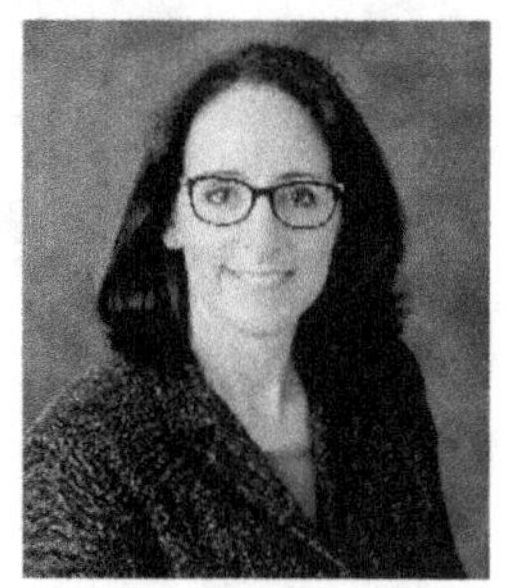

Rosemary D. Laird, M.D.

Rosemary D. Laird, M.D., graduated from Georgetown University School of Medicine in Washington, D.C. She completed a Fellowship in Geriatric Medicine and earned a Masters in Healthcare Administration.

Dr. Laird was the founding Medical Director of 'Health First Aging Services' and 'The Center for Family Caregivers' in Melbourne, Florida. She then led the development of the Memory Disorder Clinic for Advent Health Maturing Minds program in Orlando, Florida.

For over 20 years, Dr. Laird has provided specialty care for people with Alzheimer's disease and related disorders. She has been recognized as a Space Coast Humanitarian in 2011 and received the American Geriatrics Society's Clinician of the Year award in 2013.

Currently Dr. Laird is pursuing her dream of providing a new and innovative 'support system' for families facing challenges related to cognitive concerns. Check out NAN,
(Navigating Aging Needs), at **https://nanforcaregivers.com**

Rosemary Laird, M.D., is a Geriatrician and recognized expert in diagnosing and caring for patients with Alzheimer's disease.
She is an advocate for the support of family caregivers and co-authored the book Take Your Oxygen First: Preserving Your Health and Happiness While Caring for a loved one with Alzheimer's Disease.

Melissa Arnold, Founder of The BrainFlex® System
www.brainflexwellness.com

Melissa began working with seniors in 2009, as the director of an adult day program in Michigan. After moving to Orlando in 2010, she continued working in the senior care industry as a consultant, advising seniors in need of assistance in the home. Eventually, with a desire to improve the quality of care her clients received, she moved into Human Resources where she focused on recruiting caregivers who had a heart for seniors. As the Director of Human Resources, Melissa also focused on agency compliance related to AHCA and Joint Commission regulations as well as state and federal labor laws. In addition, Melissa provided on-going training for employees and education for the families of her clients. After restructuring this part of the business, Melissa was offered the position of Director of Operations, where she focused on aligning the systems and process within the business in order to provide the very best customer and employee experience. The next step for Melissa was the position of 'Executive Director', which included oversight of the Nursing Department, Human Resources, Operations, and training and development of the Sales and Marketing team. As Executive Director, Melissa led a team of directors with a focus on business development while remaining intentional in her mission to invest in the lives of her employees.

In August of 2018, Melissa made the difficult decision to resign as Executive Director of Senior Helpers in order to focus on BrainFlex Wellness Club, which she had founded in 2015. The idea for BrainFlex began in 2014, when Melissa noticed an increase in seniors experiencing dementia. It was at this time, she became a researcher of researchers, determined to find the various ways in which seniors could be proactive against age-related diseases. Her research consistently revealed the following key areas: exercise, nutrition, brain stimulating activities, social connections, prayer/meditation and sleep, as well as stress management and maintaining a positive mindset.

Once Covid-19 hit the world, Melissa began to pivot her business, offering BrainFlex sessions on-line while moving the curriculum into a series of workbooks, now referred to as The BrainFlex System. Each of the three workbook series' are designed for a specific cognitive level, with a focus on engaging the 'whole person'. Many doctors and healthcare professionals strongly encourage their patients and clients to utilize the BrainFlex system, and now we're excited to make our interactive workbooks available to seniors everywhere.

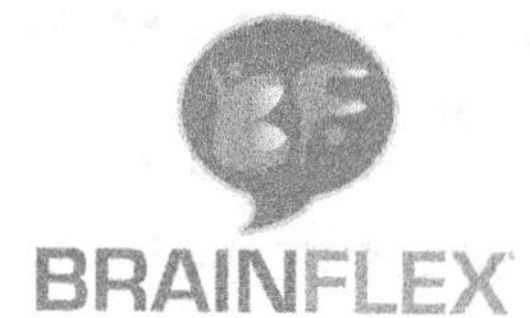

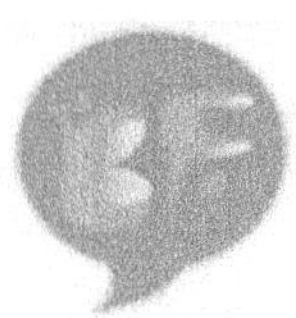

To order or reorder the next BrainFlex Workbook, or to order one of our 'Wisdom Journals', choose one of the following options:

1.) Order through the BrainFlex Wellness website. www.brainflexwellness.com

Once you're there, click on the 'WORKBOOK' tab.

On this page you will be given two choices.

A.) Order directly from amazon

B.) Save 20% by ordering directly from the BrainFlex online store.

Click on the option you prefer and follow the step by step instructions.

2.) As an alternative to the above choices, you may also send us an email requesting which series and volume(s) you would like to order, along with the number of workbooks you would like. Please send your request to:

marnold@brainflexwellness.com

NOTE: Type 'WORKBOOK ORDER' or 'WORKBOOK REORDER' in the subject line.

Once we receive your request, we will send an invoice to your email allowing you to pay for your workbook(s) directly on line. Once we receive notice of payment, your workbooks will be ordered and on their way!